The Black Woman's Guide to Breastfeeding

The Definitive Guide to Nursing for
African American Mothers

Kathi Barber

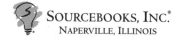

SOURCEBOOKS, INC.®
NAPERVILLE, ILLINOIS

Published by Sourcebooks, Inc.
P.O. Box 4410, Naperville, Illinois 60567–4410
(630) 961-3900
FAX: (630) 961-2168
www.sourcebooks.com

Library of Congress Cataloging-in-Publication Data

Barber, Kathi.
  The Black woman's guide to breastfeeding : the definitive guide to nursing for African American mothers / Kathi Barber.
    p. cm.
  ISBN-13: 978-1-4022-0345-9
  ISBN-10: 1-4022-0345-4
  1. Breastfeeding--Popular works. 2. Breastfeeding--United States. 3. African American mothers. I. Title.

RJ216.B27 2005
649'.33--dc22
                                        2005025004

Printed and bound in the United States of America
DP 10 9 8 7 6 5 4 3 2 1

Dedication

I would like to dedicate this book to God, who gave me the vision to help my fellow African American sisters reconnect with our breastfeeding tradition.

I would also like to dedicate this book to my husband, Noel, for his love, support, and patience with my breastfeeding passion. To my angels sent from heaven, Amyhr and Jayde, whom I breastfed with ease and with deep devotion and love.

To my mother, whom I admire for her ability to overcome any challenge with optimism and beauty. To my sister, who is the most beautiful young woman I know. To my grandma, Kat, who breastfed her four children. To Willie and Shirley, for giving birth to my husband, and for their love. To my dad, I love you.

To anyone out there supporting Black women in their breastfeeding experience, I personally thank you. Finally, I dedicate this to all my Black sisters who choose to breastfeed and experience incomparable love for their babies, who find power and confidence within the breastfeeding journey.

Acknowledgments

Special thanks to Kristen Auclair, my agent, and Deb Werksman, my editor at Sourcebooks, for giving me a chance and for making this dream a reality. Thank you to my sisters, whose inner beauty shines vibrantly, and whose support during my journey to help Black women breastfeed is immeasurable —Kim D.J., Michelle M., Michelle B., Dawn D.C., Desiree E.J., Jenise F.N., Inga T.S. (where are you?), Yvonne F., Mishawn Purnell-O'Neal, and countless others. To Beverly Spencer, who trained me, believed in me, and pointed me in all the right directions.

To my idol, Dr. Michal Young, whose advice, wit, skill, and spirit are legendary. To my breastfeeding role model, Marki Dickens, who successfully breastfed four beautiful children, and who showed me that Black women do breastfeed.

To those in the breastfeeding field who work daily to make a difference for breastfeeding mothers: to Dr. Jack Newman, for the use of his expert handouts; Kittie Frantz, for the illustrations; Karen Peters, for the use of Yellow Flags/Red Flags; INFACT Canada for the use of the risks of infant formula; the Breastfeeding Coalition of Washington/Healthy Mothers Healthy Babies Washington for the Use of the "Dear Employer" letter; and for the information on breastfeeding legislation and the International Labor Organization provided by the National Conference of State Legislatures and Congresswoman Carolyn B. Maloney.

To two special friends, Resheda Hagen of Lansinoh and Peggy O'Mara of *Mothering* magazine, whose advice and warmth is soothing to the soul.

Contents

LETTER TO THE READER FROM DR. MICHAL YOUNG ix

INTRODUCTION
Why I Wrote This Book xi

CHAPTER ONE
The Big Deal about Breast Milk: Benefits of Breastfeeding 1

CHAPTER TWO
Breastfeeding Basics 15

CHAPTER THREE
Common Concerns and Solutions: Tips for Successful Breastfeeding . . 41

CHAPTER FOUR
We Shall Overcome: Breastfeeding Barriers 79

CHAPTER FIVE
It Takes Three: Including Dad in the Breastfeeding Experience 97

CHAPTER SIX
Take the Stress Out of Going Back to Work: Plan Ahead 119

CHAPTER SEVEN
The Truth about Breastfeeding Myths 141

Chapter Eight
Our Breastfeeding Heritage.................................171

Chapter Nine
Self-Empowerment through Breastfeeding...................187

Chapter Ten
Breastfeeding Culture and Politics.......................205

Chapter Eleven
Resources for Further Support............................233

Appendix
Breastfeeding Laws by State..............................237

Bibliography.................................251

Index.................................253

About the Author.................................257

Letter to the Reader

Dear Reader,

I first met Katherine Barber in New Jersey at an April 2001 conference, "Nutrition, Breastfeeding, and Cultural Competency: Eliminating Racial Disparities in Health." We were both at this conference to speak in support of increasing breastfeeding rates, especially in the African American community. I did not get to hear her presentation, as it was later in the conference and I was only in and out for one day. However, she had a display up encouraging women to join the African American Breastfeeding Alliance. I was excited. Finally, someone had stepped into that space of vision and leadership and had taken on that daunting responsibility: tackling social forces and naysayers to tell African American women to put down that artificial milk and go back to breastfeeding.

African Americans were the last community to succumb to the subversion of the breastfeeding tradition. This lack of awareness about the benefits of human milk for human beings is truly killing us as a people. Breastfeeding not only provides optimum nutrition, but it is also a species-specific, dynamic immunological update that helps prevent colds, ear infections, pneumonia, and diarrhea in infants and children. In addition, a number of the chronic illnesses that plague us as we age—that are currently ravaging the African American community—appear to be directly related to having not been breastfed (i.e., asthma, type 1 and type 2 diabetes, hypertension, Crohn's disease, acute lymphocytic leukemia, and lymphoma). Women who do not breastfeed not only deprive their babies of good health, but they also increase their own risk for premenopausal breast cancer, epithelial ovarian cancer, and osteoporosis.

Kathi was enthusiastic and committed, brimming with the confidence that would be necessary to get the attention of women of color. She asked me if I was interested in joining the mission to make a difference. I was so honored. Finally, someone who was as interested in changing the minds of African American people about breastfeeding as I was, and more—she was willing to take that awesome step to lead. It continues to be a pleasure and an honor to work with her. She continues to lead. Sometimes this puts her in conflict with others in the breastfeeding community, who are largely our white sisters. They were initially confused, and I think sometimes not understanding that African American people need African American images and a different approach if we are to be reached. This was not a rejection of their commitment, but a need to broaden their perspectives. This process is a work in progress.

It comes as no surprise that Kathi is moving to commit to words the fire that burns inside of her; to tell African Americans that it is absolutely necessary for us to recognize that affordable and attainable health care begins with breastfeeding.

That message simply must be heard. Kathi has much to say—listen.

Michal A. Young, MD, FAAP, IBCLC
Breastfeeding Coordinator
D.C. Chapter of the American Academy of Pediatrics

Introduction

Why I Wrote This Book

It all began on March 8, 1997. At around 8:53 in the morning, after over twenty hours of painful labor, Amyhr Noel Barber was born. He looked at me calmly and I gazed at him in wonder. I latched him onto my breast, and it was the most natural experience ever.

Breastfeeding went smoothly for us for two years. It was bliss. I guess a smooth breastfeeding experience is a relative term.

When I say smooth, I don't mean it was problem-free. It's all in your perspective. I did become severely engorged. I couldn't describe to anyone the extreme pain I felt. It lasted about three days, but it seemed like weeks!

I read all that could be read on engorgement and spoke with a lactation consultant several times, but I didn't feel relief until midway through the second day. I know the sight of me was hilarious to my husband, but here's what suited me best: taking Tylenol a couple times a day and leaning over to put my breasts directly into two large bowls of very warm water several times a day. This worked better than warm compresses and a shower.

I resolved from the start that I would breastfeed, regardless of what I encountered.

Thankfully, I did not go through the trials that many women face during their breastfeeding experience, and I never thought of quitting. I figured my son deserved the best, and my breast milk was the only way he would have a jump start in life. I did not plan to breastfeed Amyhr for two years, it just happened. After three weeks, then three months, then nine months, and twelve months, I was totally hooked! I soon realized that my entire world had changed, not just because I was a mother, but because of breastfeeding. It made me take better care of my health and have a healthier diet. Breastfeeding in public didn't come easy for me. It took a long time as I am a naturally shy person. As the months progressed, I built up amazing confidence to nurse in public or even in front of visitors in our home. Breastfeeding also taught me about joy, love, and giving. I mean, I gave to my son for two years something that no one else could give him: my milk full of vitamins, minerals, antibodies, and love that all babies need and deserve. Just me. I did that for my son, and later for my daughter, too.

Breastfeeding became such a part of my life that I had to share the love with other African American women. I couldn't believe how few Black women were breastfeeding. After reading many books, taking training classes, and listening to God's purpose for my life, I began my journey to reach all of you. My hope is that this book will provide you some measure of support during your breastfeeding experience. Welcome to the joy, the love, the power of breastfeeding!

I want to share some fascinating information with you that compares our health, and the health of our babies, with other races. It will be good for you to keep these little informational gems in the back of your mind as you learn more about breastfeeding. I hope that these gems will help to strengthen your resolve to breastfeed. You and your baby are worth it.

Keep in mind:

❖ African American infants are twice as likely to die before their first birthdays as white infants.

❖ African American infants and children have the highest rate of asthma, severe asthma, and mortality caused by asthma than any other race.

❖ African Americans have a 20 percent higher occurrence of childhood obesity than white children.

❖ African American women are 2.2 times more likely to die from breast cancer than white women, and breast cancer is the second leading cause of cancer deaths of African American women.

❖ African American women are 30 percent more likely to die from ovarian cancer than white women.

Breastfeeding is an age-old remedy to these health crises, yet African American women have the lowest long-term breastfeeding rates in the country. This is more than a book about breastfeeding. It's also about providing the best start—a jump start, a head start—in life for your baby. This book can serve as a good reference point for your breastfeeding questions or concerns. You can even pass it around amongst your circle of friends to share breastfeeding knowledge.

There is no doubt you have tons of questions about breastfeeding. Doesn't breastfeeding hurt? What are the benefits of breastfeeding my African American baby? Does anyone breastfeed anymore? Isn't infant formula just as good as breast milk? If I breastfeed, won't my husband/ boyfriend be left out? How do I breastfeed? Can I continue breastfeeding when I go back to work? If this sounds like you, then reading this book will give you the answers you've been looking for.

I'm also going to share information with you about breastfeeding and its place in maternal and children's health issues—and even politics—as well as how our breastfeeding experiences compare with that of other women. The breastfeeding rates of African American women are shockingly low compared to those of Hispanic and white women. In the past ten years, our breastfeeding rates have shown some improvement, but few of us continue to provide this important form of nutrition to our babies after their six-month birthdays.

Why do we hesitate to breastfeed our babies when medical professionals across the board, from the American Academy of Pediatrics to former Surgeon General Dr. David Satcher, agree that breast milk is the best form of nutrition for all babies? I don't think we've quite realized that we have the power to breastfeed, which is like using a wonder tonic for growing healthy babies! Among other benefits, breastfeeding greatly reduces infant deaths, asthma, and childhood obesity. It helps low-birth-weight babies grow strong. What else can do that for your baby but your breast milk? Further, breastfeeding is a natural way to reduce our high incidence of mortality due to breast and ovarian cancer.

I hope you enjoy this breastfeeding handbook. It was written just for you, the African American mother, and speaks to the unique economic and social issues that may affect your breastfeeding experience. And because the success stories of Black women who have breastfeed are so inspiring, anecdotes are woven throughout this book to offer you continued encouragement and to give you real-life perspectives on breastfeeding.

Chapter One

The Big Deal about Breast Milk

Benefits of Breastfeeding

Picture this…you're at a car dealership that sells a variety of cars, ranging from economy to luxury models. You are planning to purchase a mid-range car with a down payment equal to a month's salary. You've done your research and the car you want does not fit your budget. You realize you have to settle for something you don't particularly care for, one that does not meet very high standards in safety. The salesman walks up to you and says, "Today is your lucky day. You can choose any car you want from the lot and drive it home with no down payment and the monthly car payment of your choice." After you stop laughing hysterically and realize that today is, in fact, your lucky day, you walk directly to the top-of-the-line Mercedes. It's safe. It has all the perks. It's the color you want, and the leather interior envelops you as you sit in the driver's seat.

If you have the choice of any two things—home, job, mate, meal, friend—you will absolutely choose based on quality and the ability of the particular thing to meet your needs. You'd choose a home in a neighborhood with good schools and honest neighbors. You'd work in a position that best fits your talents, goals, and financial plans. You'd find a mate you could trust and grow old with. You'd eat a meal that was delicious and healthy at the same time. You'd have a strong, dependable friend who would be there for you through good times and bad.

The point is, when you decide whether to breastfeed or give your baby formula, it's a matter of choice. Ideally, you base your decision on many factors: the best nourishment, the best start, the best protection against illness, and the best foundation for a healthy life well into childhood.

The practical and time-tested choice for giving your African American baby not just a healthy start, but also a jump start at life, is the simple act of breastfeeding.

You may be thinking, "Oh, I know the breast is best. I've heard all that." But you probably didn't know about the benefits that help to prevent many of the specific health issues that African American women—and our babies—face.

> "Human milk is uniquely superior for infant feeding and is species-specific; all substitute feeding options differ markedly from it. Exclusive breastfeeding is the reference or normative model against which all alternative feeding methods must be measured with regard to growth, health, development, and all other short- and long-term outcomes."
>
> *American Academy of Pediatrics (AAP)*

Sudden Infant Death Syndrome (SIDS)

SIDS is the unexplained sudden death of a baby from one month to one year of age. There is rarely a medical reason for the baby's cause of death in SIDS, which leaves parents and loved ones in a precarious position between mourning and looking for answers. African American infants die of SIDS twice as often as white babies do. Researchers are not sure why, but it may be because our babies tend to be born prematurely and/or with low birth weights. SIDS has also been linked to a disturbed breathing pattern in infants.

Although we don't know exactly what causes SIDS, we do know that the risk of SIDS is reduced by 50 percent if you breastfeed your baby. Part of the reason may be that breastfed babies tend to spend more time sleeping with their mothers. This allows for the mother's breathing and waking patterns to affect her baby's, helping to prevent any breathing difficulties that could lead to SIDS. Additionally, breastfeeding further decreases the risk of SIDS because breastfed babies tend to nurse often and sleep lightly, allowing them to awake more easily if they begin to have breathing difficulties. Often, babies who die from SIDS sleep deeply and soundly, have trouble trying to wake up, and may not awaken if they stop breathing.

Babies who die from SIDS have generally suffered from infections such as gastrointestinal (e.g., severe diarrhea and reflux) and respiratory (e.g., pneumonia and swelling of the baby's lungs/blocked airways). The antibodies in breast milk, as well as the immunities from your own body that are transmitted to your baby each time you breastfeed, help to protect against the infections that often lead to SIDS. So, it's not an exaggeration to say that your breast milk not only nourishes and nurtures your baby; it can actually save his or her life!

Asthma

Chances are, you have asthma, know someone with asthma, and/or know of someone who has a loved one who suffers from it. Asthma is a chronic lung disease that causes difficulty in breathing. When an asthma attack occurs, the bronchial tubes tighten and become swollen, and more mucus is produced in the airways. More than seventeen million Americans have asthma, and more than fifty-three hundred die each year because of the disease. African Americans and Latinos/Hispanics are the most susceptible to asthma. Compared to white children, our kids are four times more likely to be hospitalized due to asthma, and six times more likely to die due to complications from asthma.

A recent study shows that babies who are breastfed exclusively—fed breast milk only—for the first four months of life have a significantly lower risk of developing asthma. On the other hand, when babies under four months are given infant formula—which is made from cow's milk—they have a greater risk of suffering from asthma and related complications.

FROM ONE SISTER TO ANOTHER

When I found out I was pregnant, one of my main concerns was that asthma runs in my family. I have asthma, and a few of my cousins have had lifelong battles with asthma, with complications resulting in everything from hospitalization to surgery. One cousin even had to stop working because of constant problems from asthma. I was not breastfed, and neither were my cousins. I asked my doctor about the chances of my child developing this disease, and she told me that breastfeeding would help reduce the risk. I breastfed my son, and later my daughter. They both developed asthma, but it was very

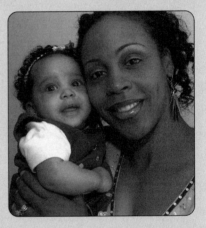

mild—fewer than one or two asthma attacks a year. My son, now six, has begun to grow out of it. All thanks to my breast milk, I think. I often wonder what would have happened to my children if I had not breastfed. Thank goodness I did!

In order to effectively prevent asthma, you should exclusively breastfeed for at least the first four to six months of your baby's life. Breast milk is full of lipids (which provide fuel), protein (which is necessary for growth and repairing tissues and cells), and vitamins and minerals. All of these are important in providing protection from disease, bacteria, and infection. Not only does breast milk help your baby to develop its own protection to fight infection, but it also transfers immunity from your body to the baby. This double-action immunity, so to speak, enhances your baby's first few years of life. If asthma happens to run in your family, as it does so often in our community, breastfeeding can help to reduce the incidents of asthmatic episodes, wheezing, and hospitalization.

Childhood Obesity

By now, nearly everyone has heard that obesity is a major health problem in this country. Between 1990 and 2000, the number of obese adults increased well over 55 percent. The greatest increase in obesity in the past twenty years has occurred in children. Today, one out of every five children is obese. Because of this alarming statistic, many health agencies and government organizations consider obesity a national epidemic. Did you know that African Americans suffer from obesity and complications due to obesity (type 2 diabetes, heart disease, high blood pressure, and cholesterol, to name a few) more than most other ethnic groups in this country? Let me give you a brief look into why we need to work hard to curb this problem.

Simply put, obesity develops when you have too much weight on your body. It is caused by many factors, including genetics (if your mother is overweight, you have a greater chance of being overweight or obese), environment (eating and exercise habits, home life), and metabolism (how many calories your body is able to burn). The good news is that obesity is highly preventable.

Breast milk contains just the right amount of fat and calories for your baby—it's unique in its makeup for your baby's individual system. There are no hidden or empty calories (those that don't benefit the diet) in your breast milk, so you can be sure that your baby will grow in an optimal manner. You might want to think of your breast milk as a natural form of weight control, not like taking Slim-Fast or going on the Atkins diet, but more of a natural, individual way to support healthy weight gain and growth. Breast milk actually helps to prevent obesity, not only in infants, but later in life as well.

Breastfeeding will help your baby to learn to do something that can help him throughout his entire life: eat until he's full, not bursting at the seams. A breastfeeding infant learns to regulate his appetite.

And get this: breast milk contains the right amount of fat a baby needs for growth, and that fat is dispensed at the right intervals for your baby's development. In essence, breast milk is not stored in the baby's system to later turn into fat. Infant formula, which is made up largely of cow's milk, is meant for an animal that will grow more than three times the size of a human at a fast rate!

About 5 percent of formula-fed babies are obese, while only 0.8 percent of breastfed babies become obese. With prolonged breastfeeding, not only can our community decrease our high rate of obesity, but we can lower our high rates of diabetes, heart disease, and a host of other illnesses that can result from being overweight.

Breast Cancer

While it's a fact that more white women have breast cancer, African American women are twice as likely to die before the age of forty from breast cancer. Why? We are often diagnosed during the late stages of the illness when treatment may not be effective. We don't receive adequate information about the importance of mammograms and breast self-exams in the early detection of breast cancer.

For each year that you breastfeed your baby, you reduce your chance of breast cancer by 4 percent. So, the longer you breastfeed and the more babies you birth, the more protection you have from breast cancer.

Scientists have found that when you are producing milk, the tissues of your breasts tend to be resistant to disease. Breastfeeding may also protect you from breast cancer because the hormones produced during this time delay the return of the menstrual cycle. Dr. Michal Young, a well-respected African American lactation consultant and breastfeeding expert, says, "Breastfeeding prolongs the time frame when there is no ovulation (like in pregnancy), therefore hormonal changes do not impact the breast continually (like during menopause)…breastfeeding has an independent protective effect against breast cancer." Someday, perhaps this protective quality of breast milk may assist in breast cancer treatment.

Breastfeeding not only provides you, the nursing mother, with protection against breast cancer, but if you have a daughter and breastfeed her, she will also be protected from breast cancer—even if she never breastfeeds her own children!

Other Important Benefits of Breast Milk
It's the Perfect Food

Breast milk is made up of at least two hundred nutrients—and many others that we don't even know about yet. It contains good fats, sugars, protein, cholesterol, vitamins, minerals, and carbohydrates—which are necessary for important things such as brain development, growth, energy, absorbing calcium into all the places it is needed, and infection protection.

It Nourishes the Body—and the Mind

Your breast milk plays an important role in your baby's brain development. Breast milk is designed with all the necessary nutrients to help your baby's brain grow in the best way possible. Infant formula is made from cow's milk. The milk of a cow is designed for the needs of a cow, and the brain development to live the life of a cow—not a human. Premature babies who are breastfed have higher IQs, on average, than premature babies who are fed infant formula. Some studies have even found that adults who were breastfed tend to have higher IQs than their peers who were not breastfed. Imagine that: providing your African American baby, who faces so many challenges as a minority, with a jump start to success.

It's Easy on the Stomach/Easy on the Bowels

Colostrum, the first milk your baby receives, helps to coat the lining of your baby's stomach. This makes digestion easy and helps to pass the meconium—baby's first stool. Breastfed babies are protected from diarrhea and constipation because breast milk is so easy for a baby's delicate stomach to digest. This first milk, along with your mature milk, is perfect for your baby's stomach. This is especially important for Black women, because more than 95 percent of African Americans are lactose intolerant and should not drink milk. Many of us suffer from gastrointestinal issues because our bodies can't break down, or have great difficulty in doing so, the lactose in cow's milk. Imagine an infant with a delicate stomach drinking infant formula. This can cause a number of stomach issues that often last into adulthood.

It Protects Babies

Each time your baby latches onto your breast, he is "re-immunized." It's not just a one-time protection. With every single feeding your baby receives throughout your entire breastfeeding experience, your baby is safeguarded. Your breast milk contains rotavirus ScIg and IgA, which are powerful antibodies that pass to your baby. In other words, your baby is protected, or has reduced occurrence, from many illnesses, including gastrointestinal diseases, pneumonia and respiratory illness (such as RSV), wheezing, ear infection, herpes simplex virus II, urinary tract infection, reflux, eczema, childhood cancer, Crohn's disease, Hodgkin's Disease, juvenile rheumatoid arthritis, and allergies. In addition to defending your baby against these ailments and diseases, breast milk helps to develop your baby's own immune system and build up his/her own protection. Breastfed babies also respond better than formula-fed babies to vaccines they receive during their early months.

It Gives Babies Better Vision and a Great Smile

Frequent feedings, which you can expect during the first few weeks, help to develop your baby's jaws and teeth. The sucking makes the muscles in the mouth strong and healthy. Breastfeeding also helps to develop your baby's eye coordination due to the switching between breasts during feedings.

Other Important Benefits of Breastfeeding for You
Lose Weight, Get Back Your Shape

Want to lose weight and return to your prepregnancy size quicker? Breastfeeding can help! This happens for two reasons. First, as a breastfeeding mother, you produce a hormone called oxytocin, which helps shrink your uterus, causing your stomach to "deflate" more quickly. Second, breastfeeding itself burns several hundred, even up to one thousand calories a day. It's almost like exercise!

More Hours in Your Day

Breast milk is always the right temperature and always ready. You don't have to sterilize bottles, find the nipple that works best for your baby, mix water with infant formula, warm the milk, test it on your wrist for temperature, or stub your toe on the dresser as you stumble down the stairs in the middle of the night to prepare a bottle.

More Money in Your Pocket

Breast milk is *free*! That's money in your pocket, bank account, child's college fund, or vacation budget. You can save anywhere from three hundred to a thousand dollars each year by not having to buy infant formula, bottles, bottle liners, and other items necessary for feeding. It can save you even more money because most breastfed babies are healthier, which means less money toward medications and other treatments for a sick baby.

Other Protection

Breastfeeding also protects you from osteoporosis, uterine cancer, ovarian cancer (a high risk in the African American community), and endometrial cancer. If you're diabetic, breastfeeding may help to decrease your insulin requirements.

More Rest for the Weary

Imagine a long labor and delivery of that baby you've been longing to meet. You finally have him in your arms. You go home and you are exhausted, and plan to rest—for a good eight hours. Then you hear bloodcurdling screams from the bassinet. You look at the clock and realize you've only been asleep for one hour. Oh! Let me be real here...less than a half hour. Junior is hungry. You groggily get out of bed to make a bottle. You and your husband repeat this process throughout the night, for weeks.

If you breastfeed your baby, you and your mate can get more rest because you can nurse while lying down. You don't have to get up to sterilize, mix, and warm infant formula. Breast milk is naturally ready and the right temperature—all the time.

Finally, Hormones That Work for You

Women who breastfeed tend to be less anxious than those who formula-feed, which is largely due to the hormones of breastfeeding.

From One Sister to Another

When I found out I was pregnant, my boyfriend left—never to return. I was left alone, bitter, and hurt. Throughout my prenatal period, though, I grew to love the baby inside. When the doctor said, "It's a girl," I looked into her eyes and felt released from a lot of the anger I felt at the beginning of my pregnancy. As I was holding her for the first time, a nurse asked, "How are you going to feed the baby?" No one had ever asked me that before. I told her that I'd use formula. The nurse smiled and talked to me about putting the baby to my breast, right there, in the birthing chair. I wasn't too sure because I had always heard it was painful. After latching my baby,

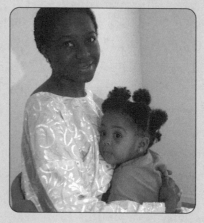

Cydney, onto my breast—it took a couple of tries—I experienced a love I didn't know I was capable of. I ended up breastfeeding her for a whole year—one of the best years of my life.

"Breastfeeding is the physiological norm for both mothers and their children. The AAFP recommends that all babies, with rare exceptions, be breastfed and/or receive expressed human milk exclusively for about the first six months of life. Breastfeeding should continue with the addition of complementary foods throughout the second half of the first year. Breastfeeding beyond the first year offers considerable benefits to both mother and child, and should continue as long as mutually desired. Family physicians should have the knowledge to promote, protect, and support breastfeeding."

American Academy of Family Physicians Policy Statement on Breastfeeding

Each time your baby latches on to your breast, two hormones are produced: prolactin and oxytocin. Prolactin tells your body to make milk, and is often called the "mothering hormone." It creates a feeling of love, making you want to be with and hold your baby more. It's also the hormone that stops ovulation. This can allow you to go several months without the return of your menstrual cycle.

Oxytocin helps your uterus to contract and prevents postpartum hemorrhaging, which can lead to infection or death. Although you don't hear about it often, there are still women in this country who die due to complications during childbirth. Oxytocin is responsible for releasing tension that may have built up from the need or desire to nurse your baby. It gives you an almost euphoric feeling, providing you a time of relaxation.

Breastfeeding can also act as a natural form of birth control, however, it may not be foolproof, and there is major room for error. Using breastfeeding as your sole source of birth control is risky, unless you plan to strictly follow the guidelines listed below. Do not let anyone lead you to believe that you won't get pregnant if you *just* breastfeed. In fact, many women get pregnant while breastfeeding, and often before their baby is a year old. Breastfeeding can be used, with extreme caution, as a form of birth control if:

❖ your menstrual cycle has not returned.
❖ your baby is not receiving any supplements, which includes water, juice, food, formula, or a pacifier.
❖ your baby is breastfeeding during the night.
❖ your baby is not sleeping through the night.

Please remember that breastfeeding as a method of birth control will not protect you from any sexually transmitted diseases.

You and Your Baby Are Worth It!

Now that you've read about some of the benefits of breastfeeding, you know just how important your breast milk is for you and your baby. It provides an unmatched start to your baby's life, with benefits that last a lifetime. Breastfeeding even helps to boost your health, too. You and your baby deserve the best life possible; and breastfeeding can be a small but vital step on the road to healthy living.

> You should not breastfeed if you are HIV positive. You may want to contact a milk bank so that your baby can still get the benefits of breast milk. Please contact a milk bank if this may be an option for you. You should also be aware that there is a significant cost associated with purchasing human milk.

Chapter Two

Breastfeeding Basics

B-day (birth, baby, breastfeeding) is approaching! No doubt you are anxiously awaiting the birth of your baby. The most important part of your success with breastfeeding is your commitment. You already have the tools—your breasts—and you'll soon have your baby. You may or may not have been reading brochures and books, learning about the technique of breastfeeding. You may understand, to some degree, how breastfeeding is supposed to work. At this point, you understand it's the best for your baby, but it is also a learning experience. For some women, breastfeeding will come almost naturally. You'll have few challenges, if any, which you seem to overcome without delay. For many women, however, breastfeeding won't be so easy. You will have problems from the very beginning and will feel like saying, "I just can't do this." Nothing will seem to be working, and on top of that, your baby may be fussy, fussy, fussy.

For all women—ones whose breastfeeding experience is relatively trouble-free, those with a bombardment of breastfeeding problems, and any in-between—breastfeeding success is based largely on your determination to make it work. Do you really want the best for your baby? Are you willing to stay the course through breastfeeding challenges? Can you find that powerful light of greatness within you to stick with breastfeeding? If you can answer "yes" to any of these questions, you will likely have breastfeeding success.

Now, what does breastfeeding success really mean? You have to determine what your breastfeeding goal is, whether it's to breastfeed for a year or longer, six months, six weeks, or six days. You already know that it's recommended for a baby to be fed only breast milk for the first six months of life, with continued breastfeeding and the inclusion of solid foods, for the next six months. But, sister, it's up to you! You have to decide what's best for you, your baby, and your situation. Don't let anyone, professional or otherwise, guilt you into making a decision to breastfeed. The longer you breastfeed, however, the better health benefits you and your baby will receive, and the bond between the two of you will be beyond compare.

What You Should Know Before the Baby Comes
Get to Know Your Breasts
As your pregnancy develops, you'll undoubtedly see changes in your breasts. They have increased in size. For some women, this is a great enhancement to your figure. For other women, however, you are not terribly excited to see your breasts grow even larger than their normal size. Don't worry: size does not matter with breastfeeding! Whether you've had tremendous growth or a modest increase, your changing breasts are a part of the experience of being a woman, which includes pregnancy and breastfeeding. Your body is preparing to feed your baby your breast milk. Certain hormones (estrogen, progesterone) are at work to get the cells and glands inside your breasts prepared for milk production.

Begin to get familiar with your breasts. Some women never touch their breasts or look at them in the mirror. It's good for you, if you haven't already, to get to know your breasts. Look at them. Touch them. Become familiar with them. This is important because you will be holding, supporting, touching, and pulling them in some fashion, for the duration of your breastfeeding experience. So, you may as well get used to being intimate with them now. You'll notice that your nipples are larger. Look at the type of nipple you have. Does it stick out? Is it flat? Does it go inward? Your nipples are important because this is *not* where you should have your baby latched.

You'll also see that the area around your nipples has increased in size. This area is called the areola, a term you'll become quite familiar with throughout breastfeeding. Prepregnancy, your areola was probably very faint in color and small in size. As your pregnancy progresses, the areola widens and darkens from pink to dark pink, from light brown to dark brown, or any variation of color in between. The point is, it will be darker and larger as your due date approaches. The areola is important because this is where your baby will latch onto your breast. You'll get more details on this later in the chapter.

You'll also see that there are raised bumps around your areola. These are called the montgomery glands, and they secrete a fluid that helps to keep your breasts clean and moisturized. You don't need to "toughen" your nipples before the baby comes. You will have colostrum for the first two to four days after you deliver. Your milk will "come in" within the first week postpartum. For some women, you will have an abundance of milk that leaks; other women may not have a lot of leaking or no leaking at all. This does not mean that you don't have milk.

Once again, each breastfeeding experience is different. You should simply get comfortable with touching your breasts, as well as talking about them. Get used to saying words like breasts, nipple, areola, suck, and latch. Go ahead. Try saying them now. You may feel silly at first, especially if you've never spoken them aloud before. By the end of breastfeeding, you'll find that saying these terms is quite easy. These are all terms associated with breastfeeding, and it's likely that at some point, you'll have to either ask a question about breastfeeding or will want to share information with a friend.

Gather a List of Resources

Support during your breastfeeding experience can help you in many ways. You can get questions answered about specific breastfeeding concerns, from sore nipples to pumping. Sometimes you may just need to hear someone say, "You're doing a great job. You can do this!" Make a list of phone numbers to call for help. Check with your physician to see if he/she has any suggestions. Contact the labor and delivery department of the hospital where you'll deliver your baby. Find out if they have a lactation consultant on staff. If so, get his/her phone number and keep it handy. Many hospitals have a "warm line" where you can call to get breastfeeding counseling by phone.

During your prenatal classes, ask about local breastfeeding support groups. Attend a meeting during your pregnancy and take a list of questions for the women who are experienced breastfeeding mothers. Talk to any of your family members, friends, or coworkers who have breastfed. Get any advice you can from them. Most cities have free parenting magazines available at grocery stores and libraries. Pick one up and look to see if there is a listing of breastfeeding resources or support groups. You may even have a chapter of the African American Breastfeeding Alliance, a breastfeeding support group; or Mocha Moms, a group of stay-at-home mothers of color. If you're on the Special Supplemental Nutrition Program for Women, Infants, and Children (WIC), let them know you're going to breastfeed and they'll likely connect you with a breastfeeding peer counselor. Check the list of resources in the back of this book for additional sources of help with breastfeeding. Look for the La Leche League (LLL) group in your area. LLL is an organization of volunteer mothers who offer skilled support and advice on most breastfeeding concerns.

Be Realistic

Your breastfeeding experience will be as individual and unique as you and your baby. No two breastfeeding experiences will be the same. No matter what people may tell you, take advice with a grain of salt and use your own instinct. What works for one mother may or may not work for you. Breastfeeding may be a walk in a rose garden for you or it may be like a roller-coaster ride. The first four to six weeks of breastfeeding can be difficult, and sometimes downright painful and frustrating. Breastfeeding is like riding a bike or roller skating: it's something that, once you get it, you'll never remember not knowing how. You're learning about your new baby and all that it takes to care for him. He's learning about this new world he's been birthed into and what it takes to voice his needs. You're both trying to figure out how breastfeeding works. His only responsibilities are to eat, sleep, cry, urinate, and have bowel movements! He's expecting that you're going to hold him or breastfeed him or change him whenever he cries. You're going to be at his beck and call. He is going to dictate your days and your nights for the first several weeks. Your responsibility is to get to know your baby, provide for his needs, and breastfeed. It's likely you'll feel like giving up. Take several deep breaths and don't give up! Look at this time as an honor and a privilege. Who else can do this, but you? Know that, regardless of the challenge, you are providing something special and unique for your baby that no one else can.

Put Your Decision in Writing

Inform your doctor or midwife that you plan to breastfeed your baby. If you create a birth plan, write it out that your baby is a breastfed baby. Make sure breastfeeding is written in your chart before you go into labor. Simply tell your doctor or the nurse in your physician's office "I am going to breastfeed and I want it written on my chart for the labor and delivery staff to see."

Also, when you get to the hospital, you, or whoever is there to support you, should notify the nursing staff that you will be breastfeeding, and that your baby should not be given any bottles or pacifiers in the nursery. Artificial nipples found on bottles and pacifiers can potentially cause a problem with your baby learning how to breastfeed. Some hospitals routinely give pacifiers in the nursery. It is important that you clearly state your baby is a breastfed baby.

It is your right to breastfeed your baby. You may feel hesitant about voicing your requirements for your baby to hospital staff. You might assume that since you're in a hospital, the staff of doctors and nurses "know best." They may know many medical procedures, but you know what's best for your baby. Begin to assume confidence about your role as a mother. Remember, you are the parent and the baby is your responsibility. If you don't feel comfortable, have your mate, husband, friend, or family member tell the staff that your baby is a breastfed baby.

How to Get Started

Breastfeed your baby right after delivery

If your delivery goes well and there are few or no complications, you should breastfeed right away. You don't need time to rest or get yourself together. Your baby won't need time to get used to the lights or the new environment. Once he is born he will naturally seek out your milk; he will likely be ready to eat right away. His sucking need will be strong in those minutes after delivery, and this is a great time to get started with breastfeeding. Why wait? If you have unexpected complications, maybe a cesarean birth, or if the baby experiences trauma, such as difficulty breathing or heart problems, then breastfeeding may be delayed. Other delays may include those that are part of the hospital policy. All hospitals will take a period of time to perform various checks (i.e., APGAR scoring) to ensure the optimal health of your baby. This may take just moments or several minutes. If you deliver in a birthing center or are attended by a midwife, you'll likely be able to nurse your baby right away. If you deliver at home, there should be no hindrance to breastfeeding right after your baby is born.

Don't send the baby to the nursery

Since breastfeeding is a learning experience, you and your baby need to be together as often as possible during those first few hours and weeks after delivery. This is key to getting breastfeeding underway quickly. If you keep your baby in the room, you begin to learn his cues without delay. You begin to zero in on his cries and what they may mean. Is he hungry, wet, sleepy, in need of love? To have a successful start at breastfeeding, you and your baby need to have lots of time to get to know each other. What better way than to have him in the room with you? Since you need to breastfeed on demand—whenever he cries—then having him in the room with you makes for a quick and easy transition into satisfying his needs. If you send your baby to the nursery, you run the risk of pacifier or bottle use, having the baby brought to you when he's screaming and agitated, and separation anxiety by either you or the baby. Any of the above can interfere with a good start at breastfeeding. Since most babies are formula-fed in the nursery, they get on a schedule; which means that your breastfed baby—who should not be on a schedule in the early months—may go for an extended period of time without eating.

Some hospitals have a policy where babies are not allowed to "room-in" with the mother. If this is the case, ask for an exception to the rule. Also, you may feel too tired or drowsy from pain medication or an epidural. If this is the case, send the baby to the nursery only during times when you feel too tired or physically unable to care for the baby in your room. If you just don't feel comfortable with keeping the baby in the room with you, or if your time in the hospital is the only time you'll get rest and relief from chores, duties, and work, then by all means send the baby to the nursery. This does not have to interfere with breastfeeding; just be sure to inform the nursery to bring the baby to you before he becomes screaming hungry. You can also call the nursery each time you are ready to feed or be with the baby. It's optimal that you keep the baby in your room, but certainly not required for breastfeeding success. The hospital provides you with diapers, wipes, blankets, and anything else you need to care for the baby while you are there. So, go ahead, keep the baby with you, and go for the breastfeeding gold!

Avoid everything but the breast

Breastfeeding gets off to its most favorable start when you don't give your baby anything but your breast. Introducing an artificial nipple found on a bottle or even a pacifier too soon can hold up, hinder, or damage the breastfeeding process. In the beginning, you don't want anything to get in the way of breastfeeding. When a baby sucks from a bottle, he gets an instant reward. The milk, be it breast milk or infant formula, pours from the hole in the artificial nipple easily. He has to put little effort into being fed. It's different with breastfeeding. Once latched onto your breast, the baby will need to suck to get milk. This requires a bit more work and energy on the baby's part. That's why it's not recommended to offer a breastfed baby an artificial nipple or bottle for about four weeks. In essence, the baby may become confused about how to get fed. If he's given a bottle, he'll come to expect instant gratification. Then when it comes time to breastfeed, he may become frustrated about having to work for his food. Some experts suggest that "nipple confusion" doesn't exist, but why rock the boat? You want this to go as smoothly as possible, especially if you're a first-time breastfeeding mom.

You might wonder: *But what if I have a c-section and I can't feed the baby for hours? Won't my baby starve?* Even if you can't feed your baby for hours, the nursery can give your baby infant formula from a cup, spoon, or syringe. This will allow your baby to be fed without the possibility of nipple confusion. *My sister says she breastfed and gave her daughter a bottle right from the start, and she never had a problem with breastfeeding.* It's not unusual for a baby to breast- and bottle-feed without any problems. In fact, many in the Hispanic community breastfeed and bottle-feed right from the start. Again, you don't want to introduce anything that could potentially get in the way of breastfeeding. You have all that your baby needs.

Get Comfortable

Before you breastfeed, get yourself into a relaxed position. If you sit in a chair or hospital bed, prop a pillow behind your back or underneath you. Any rocking chair, straight-back chair, couch, or recliner will work just fine, too. Put your feet up on a nursing stool (not required), ottoman, or a stack of books or pillows. Wear something comfortable that will give you easy access to your breasts such as a T-shirt, nursing nightgown, button-down shirt, or anything that gives you little difficulty with breastfeeding. You won't need a nursing bra. They can be helpful, but are certainly not required. Any bra will do, especially sports bras. You may also find that, if you had a c-section, a pillow placed across your stomach is helpful to alleviate any undue pressure on your abdomen. If you need help, ask your mate, husband, friend, family member, or nurse to adjust your pillow. You might even consider lying down. Either way, try to relax.

Position Your Baby

Once you are comfortable, you can position your baby. Is there a standard industry method for positioning your baby? Not really. Whatever works for optimal feeding for your baby and causes the least amount of pain for you is best; however, there are some tried and true techniques that lead to the best possible breastfeeding success. There are three main positions to hold the baby that women use during the early months of breastfeeding: cradle, football, and lying down. As your baby grows, you'll find that your breastfeeding positions will expand and vary, especially if you breastfeed your toddler. Breastfeeding while standing is not uncommon for a toddler. For the newborn, however, the way you hold and position your baby can make or break your breastfeeding experience, as well as create or reduce breast pain.

Regardless of the way you choose to hold your baby, there are a few key points about position that are vital for preventing breast pain, as well as to provide optimal breastfeeding for your baby.

❖ Keep your baby's body straight and on his side. Imagine his body as a horizontal line.

❖ Your baby's stomach should always be facing your stomach. This helps you to keep your baby's body in that horizontal line.

❖ Your baby's head should be in a straight line, facing your breast.

❖ If your baby is not on his/her side, and his body is slanted or pulling away from you, you will experience pain.

❖ If your baby's head is twisted and facing a direction other than your breast, you will feel pain, and your baby will not be able to get milk in the amount that he needs.

❖ You can help keep your baby's body straight by placing your hand on his bottom and/or thigh/leg for support.

You may find it necessary and helpful to support your breast when trying to get your baby latched. You can support your breast with the opposite hand from the arm that is supporting your baby. Take hold of your breast by placing your fingers behind, or at the back of your areola. You know that you are supporting your breast well if your thumb is on top of the breast and your other fingers are underneath your breast. You should not be touching the areola, which can put your nipple out of place in your baby's mouth. If you touch the areola while trying to support your breast, it can shift the placement of your nipple, which can lead to pain, and frustration from your baby who is trying to get milk.

It is crucial that you keep your baby's body on his side and in as straight a line as possible, with his head facing your breast, and his stomach flat against yours. Your baby will have difficulty breathing and won't be able to swallow if he's not positioned correctly. To better understand how your baby's position affects swallowing, try this. Roll saliva around in your mouth and swallow. See how easy the saliva went down? This is how easily your baby can swallow when his body is in a straight line. Now, turn your head so that you're looking behind you and swallow. See how difficult that was? This is how hard it will be for your baby to swallow if his head and body are twisted around.

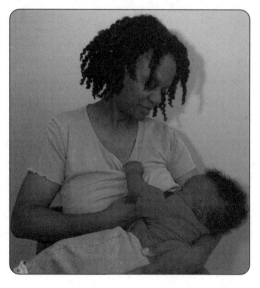

Pick up your baby and hold him so that he is resting on his side. Keep his body—head, stomach, and legs—facing you. His head should be facing your areola and lying in the crook of your arm, the place where your arm bends at the elbow. You can support his body with the same arm his head is resting in; at the same time, his bottom arm will be reaching towards your waist. You can hold his other arm, if necessary, with the opposite hand.

Football Hold

This hold actually looks like you're holding a football, and are about to run down the football field! Instead of a touchdown, your baby is getting the ultimate reward, your breast milk. This position is helpful for controlling the position of your baby's head, for women who have had a c-section

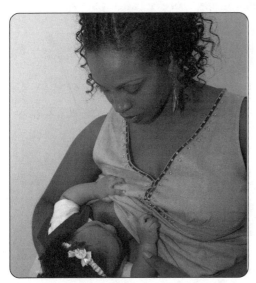

(reduces undue pressure on the stomach), and women with large breasts (helps you to see clearly when getting the baby latched). Instead of your baby being on his side in front of you, hold him at your side with his body facing upward, or him lying on his back. His body should still be straight, and his mouth should be right at your nipple. You hold his head by placing your hand at the base of his head and neck and supporting his body with your forearm. His body is essentially tucked on the side of yours. This position can be awkward to manage, but has good results once you master it.

Keys to Avoid Pain

❖ Breastfeed frequently.
❖ Be sure that your baby is latched on to the areola and not just your nipple.
❖ Position your baby correctly.

Lying Down

This position allows you to get rest, relax, and even sleep while breastfeeding. Like the football hold, it can help to alleviate any stress on your stomach if you've had a c-section. Lie down on your side in bed or on the floor, using pillows and blankets for comfort. The baby should be on his side, facing you, and his head should be at your nipple/areola area. His head can be in the bend of your arm so you can support his bottom with your hand.

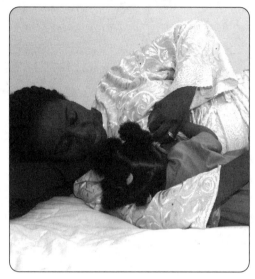

How to Get Your Baby Latched onto Your Breast

If your baby is latched on correctly, you will not experience sustained pain unless there is a complication such as thrush, or a blocked or infected milk duct. You may experience some discomfort or momentary sharp pain at the moment the baby latches on. However, once the baby is latched on and sucking, you should not feel pain. If you do, nine times out of ten it is because the baby is not latched on properly. It is worth it to take the baby off your breast at that point, and make him latch on again (details on how to do this are below). Remember, in the beginning there is a big learning curve for both you and the baby. Practice makes perfect!

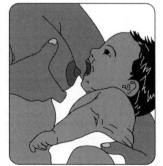

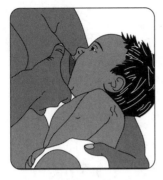

Once you get yourself comfortable, position your baby with his body and head straight, facing you, with his head right at your nipple/areola. Make sure the baby's mouth is wide open and quickly move your baby on to your breast. You can get him to open his mouth wide by rubbing your nipple against his lip. You can also squeeze a small amount of breast milk on his mouth to encourage his mouth to open. You want his mouth to open wide so that when he latches on, he is getting as much of the areola into his mouth as possible. He does not have to—and probably won't be able to—get your entire areola in his mouth. It's important that he nurses the areola, however, and not the nipple, so that his gums can squeeze the milk sinuses located beneath the areola. It may take a couple of minutes at each feeding, for him to open wide, but be patient. Also, if he's hungry, he'll be crying, which will cause his mouth to open wide. It's best, however, to get him latched on before he's screaming in hunger so you both won't get frustrated, and so you'll get a good latch.

If you are in pain, then it's possible that your baby doesn't have a good latch. You should break the latch. You can do this simply by sliding your finger, gently, into the corner of your baby's mouth. This will break the suction painlessly. If you just pull your baby off of your breast without breaking the suction, you will experience severe pain, and possibly nipple damage.

Your nipple should be far back in your baby's mouth. Both of your baby's lips should be turned outward (picture a duck's lips, those of a fish, or two Pringles potato chips back to back). His top lip should be in the direction of the top of your areola, and the bottom lip should be in the direction of the bottom of your areola. Both lips should be reaching toward the back of your areola, away from the direction of your nipple. His lips should not be tucked or sucked inward. If either lip is curved inward, or it looks like he is sucking on his top or bottom lip, break the latch and start over. If his lips are tucked in instead of flared out, he won't be able to effectively compress the milk sinuses beneath the areola. You will know that your baby has a good latch if:

❖ you don't feel pain (although there may be some discomfort until you get the hang of it, you should not be in excruciating pain).

❖ your baby's lips are flanged outward, like fish or duck lips.

❖ your baby's tongue is tucked under your breast.

❖ you hear a deep swallowing sound from your baby.

❖ you do not see dimples in your baby's cheeks.

How to Break Your Baby's Latch

It's easy! Slide your finger gently into the corner of your baby's mouth and break the suction. Do not pull your baby off your breast without breaking the latch. If you do, you will experience pain, and may injure your nipple.

How Breastfeeding Works

The amount of breast milk you produce is based on supply and demand. The more you breastfeed your baby, the more milk you'll be able to produce, and the more abundant your milk supply will be. This is why it's so important for you to breastfeed as soon as possible after the birth of your baby, and breastfeed on demand, or as often as your baby needs. You've probably heard someone say, "I couldn't breastfeed because my milk dried up," or "I just didn't have any milk." It's likely that she didn't breastfeed her baby as often as necessary. It's rare for a woman not to produce breast milk. Even women who have never become pregnant can breastfeed. Your breasts are made up of a complex system of parts that work together with your baby to produce breast milk.

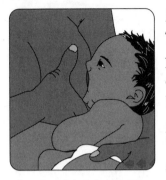

Nipple

The place where your breast milk is sent out to your baby's mouth. When your baby is latched on correctly, your nipple will be stretched far back into your baby's mouth, and rests in the soft palate area. When you hear women say that "breastfeeding hurts," it's likely that the baby was sucking the nipple and not the breast. Your nipples shouldn't hurt. You can test where the soft palate is and just how soft that area is when your baby is latched on well. Beginning at the front of your mouth, slide the tip of your tongue on the roof of your mouth as far back as it can go. Do you feel that soft, squishy area? That's where your nipple will be when your baby has a good latch. Your *nipple* does not have milk pooled inside of it, so when your baby latches there, he can become frustrated because he'll be getting a small amount of breast milk. If this lasts for

---

Pain Check

If you feel discomfort or are mildly uncomfortable, you are learning and probably on your way to breastfeeding success. Pain, however, is a clear warning signal that something is probably wrong. If you feel pain, check and correct the following:

❖ Is your baby nursing your nipple?
❖ Are your baby's lips turned inward?
❖ Are you holding your baby too far away from you?
❖ Is your baby's body or head turned away, instead of towards you?

For more information on thrush, plugged ducts, and other breastfeeding concerns, please see pages 41 to 76.

too many days, he could actually fail to gain the weight he needs for optimal health. Also, the more your baby is latched onto your nipple, the more pain you'll experience, and this could ultimately lead to sore, cracked, and/or bleeding nipples. You can still breastfeed if this happens, but it'll be more painful until your nipples heal. You may even give up.

Areola

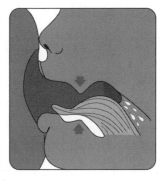

The brown area around your nipple. The areola is the key to an effective latch and feeding. It's also important because, if your baby is latched on to your areola correctly, you won't have the pain that comes if your baby is latched on to your nipple. Your breast milk is collected underneath or behind (under the layers of skin and fat tissues) the areola. When your baby is latched onto the areola, he can effectively suckle and get the milk out of your breasts, which leads to healthy weight gain and a more satisfied baby.

Sinus

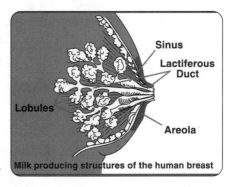

Located beneath your areola. This holds the milk after it travels from the milk ducts.

Alveoli

Inside the breast, near the chest wall. This is where the breast milk is actually produced.

Ducts

Connects the alveoli and sinuses. The ducts are passageways that allow the milk to travel from the alveoli to the sinuses.

How Your Breasts and Your Baby's Mouth Make Breast Milk

Each time your baby breastfeeds, the process of making breast milk begins. People think that breast milk is just sitting there in the breasts, waiting for a baby to suckle. This is part of the reason why so many people think that breast milk can dry up and spoil. Your breasts are not like a water system, where all you have to do is turn the faucet on and the water pours out. When your baby latches onto your breast, signals are sent to the pituitary gland in your brain, which say, "make milk." This message kicks in the production of prolactin, a hormone that starts making milk.

Once milk is made in the alveoli, a second hormone, oxytocin, releases the milk—a feeling of tingling in some women—and it flows down into the milk sinuses. At the same time milk is being made and sent to your baby, the hormones are telling your ovaries to "stop ovulating," which creates a limited natural protection against pregnancy. This all happens

IS MY BABY GETTING ENOUGH MILK?

You can feel confident that your baby is getting enough breast milk if your newborn:

❖ nurses at least every two hours (that's two hours from the beginning of feeding to the beginning of the next feeding).

❖ suckles for twenty minutes or more on one or both breasts.

❖ has six to eight wet diapers and two to five bowel movements a day.

❖ is gaining weight.

each time your baby latches onto your breasts. You can see now why the amount of breast milk you make is based on how often you breastfeed your baby. Your breasts aren't just manufacturing milk, awaiting your baby to feed, instead breast milk is made once your baby latches on to you. As long as you're breastfeeding your baby often and on demand, particularly in the early weeks and months, you should be able to provide the milk that your baby will need.

Your baby will also breastfeed more often when he's going through a growth spurt, which will, in turn, increase the amount of breast milk to provide the nutrients he needs. Once the growth spurt has passed, your breast milk will level out to what your baby needs. This is one of the many advantages of breastfeeding because you always have enough milk, and it's always ready because you and your baby dictate how much milk there will be.

Ingredients in Breast Milk

You read a lot about breast milk, how it's the best for your baby, but why? What makes breast milk so perfect for your baby's needs? For one, there are natural and incomparable ingredients that make breast milk the best choice for all babies. It contains the following for your baby's best nutrition:

Water

Breast milk is made up of about 87 percent water, and is important for keeping your baby hydrated.

Fats (lipids)

Your baby will receive a large portion of his calories from fat. DHA (docosahexaenoic acid) and AA (arachidonic acid) are fatty acids. Both DHA and AA work to give your baby optimal brain and visual development. It's that special component of breast milk that will increase your baby's IQ.

Protein (casein, whey, lactoferrin)
Protein helps to provide energy and assists in the reduction of iron deficiency and resistance against infection.

Carbohydrates (lactose)
Carbohydrates help your baby to absorb calcium and supply energy to your baby's brain.

Nucleotides
These compounds play a major role in the development of your baby's ability to fight disease, as well as the development of his gastrointestinal system.

Vitamins
Breast milk contains vitamins A, D, E, and K in the amounts your baby needs. There are some instances, however, when your pediatrician may suggest that you give your breastfed baby vitamin D supplements. The American Academy of Pediatrics now suggests that breastfed babies be given vitamin D supplements to prevent rickets, a bone disease that results from a severe vitamin D deficiency. This is often due to either a severe lack of vitamin D in the mother's diet or if the baby is never exposed to sunlight (a natural and often effective means of acquiring adequete amounts of the vitamin). Rickets is often seen in mothers who have darker skin tones, and in babies of darker skin tone. If you are uncomfortable with giving your baby supplements, you can talk with pediatrician about continued use of your prenatal supplements while your breastfeeding, safe ways to expose your baby to sunlight, and/or including vitamin D in your diet.

Minerals

Breast milk contains a small, but adequate, amount of iron, and prevents the risk of overload. Too much iron can cause constipation, stomach pain, and the potential to break down the amount of immunity that lactoferrin helps to create. After your baby is six months old, doctor's recommend iron supplements by way of iron enriched cereals, vegetables, and/or meats.

Other minerals in good supply are calcium, potassium, sodium, magnesium, copper, selenium, chromium, manganese, zinc, molybdenum, and nickel.

Antibodies

The immunological aspect of breast milk makes it all the more incomparable. It provides immunities against diseases and illness that can severely harm, or even prove deadly to, an infant. Not only do you pass your immunity from disease to your baby through your breast milk, but your breast milk also helps to strengthen your baby's own ability to fight disease.

Colostrum

Babies receive colostrum for the first three to five days of life, or until their mother's milk comes in during the first week. Colostrum is your baby's first immunization. It is full of disease-fighting antibodies, which protect your baby from many illnesses, including diarrhea, gastrointestinal issues, ear infections, pneumonia, and other respiratory viruses. It is thick and has a yellowish color and is often called "liquid gold." It is easily digestible, and coats your baby's stomach so that he can pass the meconium, his first stool. Some women think that this yellowish fluid they see is not breast milk and will not be sufficient for their baby. However, colostrum is highly concentrated with all the vitamins, minerals, fats, protein, calcium, and antibodies your baby will need. It is sufficient and optimal for your baby's health while you await your mature milk.

How to Know if Your Baby is Getting Enough Milk

There's no real way to measure the exact amount of breast milk you have, but there are a few things you can keep track of to be sure your baby is getting enough breast milk. It also help to keep a breastfeeding log during your few weeks of breastfeeding. Keep a notepad handy, along with all your baby's essentials—diapers, wipes, etc.—and write down the times of each feeding, how long your baby nursed, and the number of wet and soiled diapers for each twenty-four-hour period. These notes will help you keep track of your feedings and the amount of diapers your baby has a day. You know that your baby is getting enough breast milk if:

❖ **You are breastfeeding your baby at least every two to three hours a day; that's at least twelve times in each twenty-four-hour period.** More likely, you'll be breastfeeding every hour, which generally lasts for the first few weeks, and during times when your baby is experiencing a growth spurt (around the second and sixth weeks, and again at three months). You should not let your breastfed newborn sleep for longer than a three-hour period because he may be missing valuable nutrients during feedings he needs for growth. At first, he won't always wake up for a feeding, so get used to waking him up to breastfeed. If you find that you have a sleepy baby, you can do a number of things to wake him, such as change his diaper, remove his clothes, tickle his feet, or run your fingers gently down his back. Breast milk is digested quickly: your baby will need to refuel frequently. So no schedule for your breastfed baby. You should be feeding on demand, or anytime you or your baby wants. Frequent feedings increase your milk supply, and prevent discomfort.

❖ **You are not in pain.** When you're in pain, that's a signal that your baby isn't latched on well. If your baby is not latched on correctly, he will not be able to get the amount of breast milk he needs. If you feel

WARNING SIGNS

Seek help from a breastfeeding peer counselor, lactation consultant, or your physician if:

❖ your newborn is sleeping for long periods of time, over three hours.

❖ you have consistent problems with your baby's latch.

❖ your baby only breastfeeds for a couple of minutes on each breast.

❖ you are in pain.

❖ after day five, or a few days after your milk comes in, your baby is having less than six wet diapers and three soiled diapers.

❖ your baby is not producing any wet diapers.

❖ your baby does not seem to be full or satisfied after several feedings.

pain, break the latch and start again. This may seem tedious, but it's for the benefit of you and your healthy, growing, breastfed baby.

❖ **Your baby seems satisfied, sleepy, or full after breastfeeding.** Your baby should breastfeed for at least ten to fifteen minutes (or longer) on each breast per feeding, although this is not an exact science. It ensures, however, that your baby gets to the hind milk, which is the fattier milk that's produced at each feeding. The milk your baby gets during the first few minutes of feeding is the foremilk, which is thinner and contains less fat. The hind milk is richer in color and contains the fat your baby needs. The breast milk production process begins when your baby latches on, but it can take up to five minutes to get flowing. You may feel a tingling sensation in your breasts. This is known as the let-down or the "milk ejection reflex" (MER) and signals that your milk will soon be flowing quickly to your baby. Don't be concerned if you don't

How to Express Milk with Your Hand

Have your milk storage container ready. Wash your hands. Gently massage your breast in a circular motion. Hold your breast in your hand with your thumb on top, behind your areola and away from your nipple, and your other fingers beneath your breast. Push and squeeze your fingers backwards, towards your chest. You should be able to feel your milk sinuses behind your areola. Repeat. Once you begin to see your milk pouring out, you've probably got it right.

feel the let-down, because some women do not experience this sensation. Whether you feel the let-down or not, your breasts should feel markedly empty or soft after a feeding. After you and your baby get into a breastfeeding rhythm, you may be able to switch between breasts based on the feeling of your breasts being emptied of breast milk—from full of milk to being deflated so to speak—as opposed to how long your baby has been nursing; but in the beginning, it can be helpful to use this "time frame" as a guide. By all means, do what works for you and your baby!

❖ **Your baby produces one to two wet diapers during the first few days of breastfeeding.** This is normal. On the first day or two, his stool will be thick, tarry, and black. Then as breastfeeding is established, you should expect your baby to have at least six to eight wet diapers, and two or more stools a day. You should know that your breastfed baby's bowel movements will look different than a formula-fed baby's. It will be yellowish in color, loose, and seedy in consistency. It will look like yellow diarrhea.

❖ **Your baby is gaining weight, about one pound a month or four to six ounces a week.** Most physicians, health care providers, and insurance agencies require that breastfed babies have a pediatrician visit within the first week of birth. By seeing that your baby is gaining weight well, you can be reassured that breastfeeding is working. If counting diapers doesn't satisfy you, you should feel free to drop in at your pediatrician's office. The nurses should be open to weighing your baby.

How Do I Know if My Baby is Hungry?

- ❖ Breastfeeding early and frequently will help you to begin to understand your baby's cues.
- ❖ Your baby will actually turn his head from side to side with his mouth open, looking for your breast. It's called rooting—nature's way of getting you and your baby in sync with each other.
- ❖ Your baby may move his arms and legs, or attempt to place his hands or fingers in his mouth.
- ❖ Of course, crying is a good signal. You'll soon learn the difference between the cry of "I'm hungry" and "I want you to hold me" and "I need a diaper change."

Chapter Three

Common Concerns
and Solutions

Tips for Successful Breastfeeding

Problem: Sore Nipples—including cracked and/or bleeding nipples

This is usually related to a baby who is not latched on the right way, or who is positioned improperly. It can also be related to thrush. Sore nipples are common during the early weeks of breastfeeding, during any time that your baby is experiencing a growth spurt, or even during teething.

Your Emotions

You may feel like crying and think, "I can't go through another feeding." This is absolutely normal. The good news is that you can make it through this. Take it one feeding at a time, and feel confident that it can be corrected by paying attention to a few simple details.

Solution

Don't stop breastfeeding! You can still breastfeed if your nipples are cracked and bleeding. It may be painful, but it's best to keep breastfeeding. Continued and more frequent feeding will actually help reduce nipple soreness. Remember to have your baby nurse the areola and not the nipple. Check to be sure that the baby's body is straight and facing you. His head should not be twisted away from your breast. His mouth should be opened wide when you pull him quickly to your breast. One of the simplest remedies for sore and/or cracked nipples is breast milk itself. Squeeze a small amount from your breast and rub it onto the cracked area. Allow it to air dry. Some cultures use breast milk to treat pinkeye and eczema of the skin.

Quick Tips

- Keep breastfeeding.
- Breastfeed on demand, not on a schedule.
- Breastfeed on the least painful side first.
- Check your baby's position and latch.
- Go topless! Allow your nipples to air dry without a bra or other clothing. This allows for more skin to skin bonding with your baby, and your nipples will heal more quickly.
- In cases of extreme pain, as long as it's *not* caused by a blocked duct or by thrush, you may purchase breast shells. These are soft cups with air holes that are worn inside your bra. They allow air to get to your nipples, which aids in healing, and it keeps your bra and other clothing from rubbing and further irritating your nipples. These can be purchased at your local hospital or drugstore. Remember, extreme pain is a red flag that something is not quite right with breastfeeding. Please check for correct latch, position, white patches on your baby's mouth (thrush), or other red flags discussed in chapter 2.
- Place some of your breast milk (squeeze out some with your hand) on the nipples.

❖ Use Lansinoh cream. This is a pure, safe, thick lanolin cream that can help in soothing and healing your sore and cracked nipples. Lansinoh is completely safe to use, and your baby can breastfeed even if you've just placed the cream on your nipples. Lansinoh can be purchased at any drug store, or other stores where baby items are sold.

❖ Don't use soap or other harsh agents on your breasts, which can lead to additional dryness and cracking.

❖ Before and during a feeding with sore nipples, try to relax and think about how important your breast milk is for your baby. Take a deep breath and meditate on something soothing and relaxing.

❖ Be patient! Sore nipples should only last a few days.

Problem: Engorgement

You know that your breasts are engorged if: your breasts feel swollen, hard, and/or warm; you feel extreme pain; your nipples are flatter than usual; your baby is having a hard time latching on; or your breasts appear red. Engorgement happens during the first few days of your milk coming in because there is an increase in the blood flow in your breasts. It can last for one to three days. Engorgement will also happen during times that your normal breastfeeding is interrupted; for instance, if either you or your baby is sick and there are less feedings. Any time that your breasts stop making the amount of milk they normally do, engorgement may occur. If you begin to skip feedings or miss a pumping at work, you will probably feel engorgement. It may not always be as painful as in the early days, but you'll notice a difference in your breasts.

Your Emotions

There's no doubt that engorgement makes many women want to give up. It's painful. You're frustrated. And your baby doesn't seem satisfied. Your breasts have doubled or tripled in size and you can't see any way past painful feedings. You can't even imagine having to place your baby onto your breasts. The thought of another feeding makes you cringe! That infant formula you have for "just in case" starts looking really tempting. This is all normal. Your feelings are completely justified. Just hang in there. If you can give birth and endure the pain that it often creates, you can make it through a couple days of discomfort. Again, take this one feeding at a time. Keep telling yourself, "I am providing the best for my baby. No one else can do this but me. I am a powerful mother with liquid gold for my baby."

Solution

Don't stop breastfeeding! This is important so that your baby can get the milk out of your breasts and begin to regulate the amount of milk your breasts are producing. With continued feedings, the blood flow to your breasts will balance out and you'll begin to feel relief. It should only last twenty-four to forty-eight hours.

Quick Tips

❖ Nurse frequently and try to empty your breasts at each feeding.

❖ Massage your breasts with your hands or use a breast pump to release some of your breast milk. This will help to soften your areola and allow your baby to latch on with less difficulty. You can also do this after a feeding for additional relief.

❖ Use warmth to soften your breasts before a feeding. Stand in a warm shower and let the water soothe your breasts. Place a cloth or towel warmed with running water on your breasts. Place dry rice in a cotton sock and warm in the microwave for a few seconds, just until warm, not hot. Use this soft pack to help soften your breasts.

❖ Use cold compresses to reduce swelling. An icepack or a bag of frozen vegetables placed in a towel works well.

❖ Use cabbage leaves. Peel leaves from a fresh head of green cabbage and place around the breasts, inside of your bra. Keep the cabbage leaves there until they wilt. Then remove. Do not leave the cabbage leaves there for an extended period after they wilt because it may begin to decrease your milk supply.

Problem: Plugged Ducts

These are lumps you may notice in your breasts. Plugged ducts happen when the flow of milk through one or more of your milk ducts is blocked. You may have plugged ducts if you feel lumps in your breasts, even near or under your arm. You may think the following suggestion is unreasonable and downright impossible. However, if you're suffering from painful plugged ducts, chances are you'll try this solution to find some relief.

Here it goes: Get more rest! Stop what you've been doing—entertaining, cooking meals, doing laundry—and slow down. Often, plugged ducts, as well as engorgement and other breastfeeding problems, are caused by lack of rest and a fast return to pre-baby activities. This happens because it's likely that you are busy around the house or start to move back into your usual routine too quickly, before breastfeeding is sufficiently established; and you may not be breastfeeding as long as you should. Paying more attention to breastfeeding and resting can help you to recover from and prevent plugged ducts, and a host of other breastfeeding problems. So stop, take a rest, and breastfeed your baby. You may not get this opportunity to relax in rest mode for a long time!

Your Emotions

You may feel confused about breastfeeding and wonder, "What's wrong with my breasts?" You may even think that the lump is related to cancer. Many women who've never breastfed, and who don't give themselves monthly breast exams, are unfamiliar with their breasts and how they feel. Your breasts should return to normal within a day or so.

Solution

Keep breastfeeding! This should go away within two days, and you'll feel relief with frequent breastfeeding.

Quick Tips

❖ Use heat between feedings. Apply a warm compress to the lump before you breastfeed. Stand in a very warm shower and allow the water to soothe the affected breast. Use the rice sock mentioned earlier. Fill a bowl with warm water and soak your breast(s) in there.

❖ Massage the lump. Start by gently using your fingertips to massage the lump towards the top of the breast and keep massaging as your fingers travel down towards your nipple. Do this in a circular motion until you feel some relief. You can do this between and during feedings.

❖ Allow your baby to feed from the breast with the lump first.

❖ Breastfeed often.

❖ Get rest and try to relax. Use the lying-down position while breastfeeding.

Problem: Mastitis

Mastitis is a breast infection. It can sometimes start as a plugged duct. It can also be caused by too many skipped feedings, incorrect latch/position, and stress you may be experiencing. Your breasts may feel hot, swollen, and/or red. You are undoubtedly in a great deal of pain. You may also feel like you have a cold or experience flu-like symptoms and have a fever.

Lack of rest is a major culprit in creating an environment for breast infections. This is not to say you will get eight hours of sleep a night, because, let's face it, that's not going to happen for a few months yet. However, you should be sleeping and/or resting. Sleep when your baby is sleeping. It's tempting to squeeze in several chores and other activities while your baby is asleep. Try to resist this temptation to get things done. The things you feel need to get done can generally wait. A few dishes in the sink and a growing laundry pile are not that big of a deal. If you're worried about what people will think when they come to visit, remind yourself and others that your role as a mother and a breastfeeding mother is fundamentally more important than a perfectly clean house. Rest helps to calm your mind and emotions, as well as rejuvenate you for successful breastfeeding.

Your Emotions

You probably feel like you're going to pass your infection on to your baby. Since breast milk is full of living blood cells, your baby is given immunity to illnesses you may experience. Breastfeeding is not only safe while you have a breast infection, it's also necessary to keep your baby fed, to prevent severe engorgement, and to keep you emotionally sure that you're providing the best for your baby, even when you're sick. You may feel stressed with all the responsibilities of being a mother and taking care of your baby. This is normal. You should know that things will balance out, but that you must take care of yourself and get rest to keep your emotions stable.

Solution

Keep breastfeeding, and contact your physician. A breast infection is often, although not always, treated with antibiotics prescribed by your doctor. A word of caution: Your physician, and other well-meaning friends and family, may tell you that you need to stop breastfeeding to treat the infection. This is simply not true, and generally comes from a lack of breastfeeding education on your physician's part. If your doctor advises you to stop breastfeeding, contact a lactation consultant in your area and get a second opinion. This may seem drastic, but many, many women have had their breastfeeding experiences ruined because they've been told to stop breastfeeding. If you have a breast infection, your baby has already been exposed. Sudden weaning will exacerbate the infection, aggravate your emotions, and traumatize you and your baby.

Quick Tips

❖ Keep breastfeeding, but breastfeed on the less painful side first. By nursing on the least painful side, it can give the damaged/sore breast more time to heal, causing less pain. This doesn't mean to not nurse on that breast, just nurse on the other side first, until healing takes place.

❖ Gently massage your breast.

❖ Use heat for comfort.

❖ Take time to rest. Rest plays an important role in the treatment of mastitis and other breast infections. If you're back to work, this is a good time to take a sick or personal day off. If you're at home, ask your spouse, partner, family member, or friend for additional help around the house. If possible, arrange for someone to pick up any other children from school.

Problem: Thrush

This is a yeast infection in your baby's mouth, which spreads to your breasts. Your nipples may itch, burn, be sore with some shooting pain during feedings, and/or become pink in color. You will see white patches inside your baby's mouth and on his tongue. You may also notice redness in his diaper area. It is sometimes caused by antibiotic use.

Your Emotions

When you see white patches in your baby's mouth, especially after breastfeeding has been going well for a period of time, don't panic. Thrush is easily treated and prevented.

Solution

Don't stop breastfeeding. Frequently replace nursing pads, because yeast flourishes in warm, wet places. Keep your bras clean. Give your nipples ample time in fresh air—go topless or braless.

Quick Tips

❖ Contact your doctor. Thrush needs to be treated with an antifungal cream for your breasts and drops for your baby's mouth, prescribed by your doctor. Take the medicine as indicated, and complete the entire course of treatment.

❖ Wash and boil for five minutes or so any items that came in contact with your breasts or baby's mouth during infections, such as pacifiers, bottle nipples, teething toys, breast shells/shields, or parts to a breast pump. If you don't, these items can reinfect you and the baby, causing a new cycle of thrush.

Other Concerns

Normal experiences, emotions, and behaviors that you have about breastfeeding your baby are areas that you can overcome by reading breastfeeding literature and/or speaking with a breastfeeding peer counselor, lactation consultant, midwife, or your doctor.

Prenatal Concerns
Previous Breast Surgery

As long as your milk sinuses or ducts were not damaged during the surgery, breastfeeding should not be a problem. Talk with your physician and/or surgeon to find out if your areola was damaged.

Previous Lactation Failure

Each breastfeeding experience, like each pregnancy, is different. If you didn't have a successful experience breastfeeding in the past, you can start fresh. Examine why you didn't have success, and see what you can do differently. Anytime your baby is latched on and receives milk, you have success at breastfeeding.

Flat or Inverted Nipples

If your nipples are flat or inverted, you may experience a little more of a challenge with getting breastfeeding off to a good start. This is not universal though, and just because you have flat or inverted nipples, that does not mean you will have breastfeeding challenges. If you find difficulty in getting your baby latched, try stimulating your nipples so that they protrude by using your fingers or pumping before a feeding. You can also wear breast shells inside your bra, which aid in bringing out your nipple.

Disabled Mother

You can still breastfeed. You may need additional help with positioning, but breastfeeding should not be a problem.

Breast Changes

Some women experience more breast changes than others. Your breasts may grow a lot or may not grow much at all during your pregnancy. This has nothing to do with breastfeeding. You can sufficiently feed your baby regardless of your breast size or lack of breast change during pregnancy.

Maternal Concerns

Excessive Fatigue

It is normal to be exhausted during your early weeks of breastfeeding. You are responsible for filling all the needs of your baby, from breastfeeding to nurturing to changing diapers. You are working hard to care for your baby, not to mention any other siblings, and a husband or boyfriend. It's likely that you're skipping meals because you haven't figured out yet how to eat while breastfeeding or how to tend to your own nutritional needs. You might also have had a traumatic delivery and are taking pain relievers, which can cause you to feel fatigue.

Don't be supermom! It's an overrated and often overwhelming experience. If someone offers you help, say yes! When you have company, ask them to help fold laundry while you're talking. Ring up a friend and ask for dinner to be brought over for your family. Get your mate to help around the house. Eat between feedings, even if you're not hungry. You need to keep up your calorie intake so that your body will replenish itself after feedings. Also, you need all those nutrients to keep your energy flowing. Keep quick snacks handy, such as granola bars, fresh fruit, and vegetables that you can eat on the run. Drink plenty of water and other fluids to stay hydrated. Finally, don't get up for those first six weeks. Once people see you moving about, it will be assumed that you've got things under control and it's business as usual. Even if you're dying to get moving, try to rest as long as you can because responsibilities are simply awaiting your return.

Mild Depression

Feeling blue after you have a baby is normal. It usually lasts for a few weeks postpartum. It's caused by many things, such as unbalanced hormone levels, sleepless days and nights, a letdown from the excitement of the baby's arrival, fear about your role as a mother, as well as any stress you already have going on in your life. You may feel like crying one minute, then laughing the next. You may be hungrier than normal, or you may find that you don't have an appetite. These feelings should subside within a few days to a couple of weeks. Lots of rest can help you feel more able to deal with your emotions. Sleep when the baby sleeps! Seek support and help from loved ones and friends. Talking about your feelings to other moms can be a big help during this time. Know that these feelings will pass and you'll begin to feel like your old self, or your new self, soon.

Need for Prescription Drugs

While many medications are safe to take while breastfeeding, be sure to contact your doctor. He may suggest that you stop breastfeeding because you

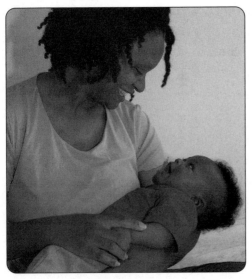

need to take a certain drug. If this is the case, ask your doctor to research alternatives. You should also contact a lactation consultant, or go online to see if there are alternatives to the medication he/she has recommended. Often, doctors are not educated about breastfeeding, and to be safe, they'll suggest that you stop nursing. It's generally better for a mother to be treated with a different medication and continue breastfeeding than to stop breast-feeding, which leaves her baby open to disease, and may make her feel guilty.

Family History of Allergies

It's likely that allergies to the environment (dust, mold, ragweed, etc.) or foods may be inherited by any baby. This should not interfere with breastfeeding.

Infant Concerns

Jaundice

This means that your baby has more bilirubin than needed and his liver is trying to break down the extra blood cells. You may notice that your baby's eyes and skin have a yellowish tint, a tell-tale sign of jaundice. Many babies experience jaundice during the early weeks after birth and it goes away within a few weeks. Some babies, however, will need treatment. Breastfeeding should still be continued if your baby needs treatment for jaundice. If your baby is jaundiced, you may notice that he is very sleepy. This is normal, but you will need to wake him more frequently for feedings. Often, babies will be placed under special lights in the nursery or treated with phototherapy to bring down their bilirubin levels. If the jaundice continues past three weeks, you should contact your pediatrician.

Diarrhea/Vomiting

The stool of a breastfed baby is very different from that of a formula-fed baby. Your breastfed baby's stool will be loose, mucous-y, and yellowish in color. You may think that he has diarrhea. This is not the case. In fact, breast milk is so easily digested that your baby probably will have frequent bowel movements. Some mothers think that breastfed babies don't vomit. All babies vomit from time to time, some more than others. As long as your baby is gaining weight, and not projectile vomiting (where the vomit shoots out forcefully), then your baby is doing fine.

Weight

You should count your baby's diapers (six to eight wet diapers and two to five soiled diapers a day) to be sure he's getting enough breast milk. If you find that your baby is making fewer wet and soiled diapers a day and he is slow to gain weight, you should increase your feedings. Offer the breast as often as possible. Be sure that your baby is latched on properly, positioned well, and is nursing until your breasts feel empty, so that he can get to fattier milk that comes toward the end of breastfeeding.

Premature Baby (after Thirty-Four Weeks)

Breast milk is best for a premature baby. The milk of a mom who gave birth prematurely is made especially for that premature baby, and can help the baby get to a desired weight more quickly. Skin to skin contact is also beneficial for the health of a premature baby. You may have to pump your milk and bring it to the hospital if your baby stays there after you are discharged. Breastfeeding can help you to feel more connected with your baby, especially if you're separated for a period of time. Premature babies sometimes have difficulty with sucking. This will require more commitment from you, and maybe assistance from a breastfeeding professional. A Supplemental Nursing System may also help if your baby has a difficult time sucking.

Colic

Colic is the diagnosis for a baby who cannot be satisfied, seems to be in pain, and cries for extended periods of time (at least three times a week, from a few minutes to two or more hours, especially at nighttime). The fact is, researchers don't have much information on colic and why babies suffer from it. What they have found is that colic:

❖ affects 10 to 20 percent of all babies.

❖ starts by the time a baby is about three weeks old.

❖ may last for a few weeks.

Colic may be caused by: restlessness, overstimulation, stress, an undeveloped digestive system, severe hunger, and stomach distress from foods in the mother's diet. You may notice colicky behavior after you've had cow's milk, broccoli, caffeine, nuts, cabbage, or wheat. You may want to stay away from any food that seems to upset your baby, or enjoy these foods when you won't have to nurse for several hours. You should continue breastfeeding a colicky baby because it will help to soothe him. He may want to breastfeed all the time. Well meaning family, friends, and even your doctor may tell you that you should stop breastfeeding, or that your breast milk is causing the colic. This is simply not the case. Breastfeeding does not cause colic.

You can help to calm a colicky baby by giving warm baths and playing soft music in a darkened room. Rock the baby gently. You can wrap him snugly in a blanket, with his arms pinned to his sides. This is called swaddling. Carry him in a sling, Snugli, or other infant carry device. Take him for a car ride, etc. Massage, with care, your baby's back. Be extra diligent with burping, which may help if your baby's colic is related to his digestive system. Coping with a colicky baby is challenging. You may feel like you're going to lose your mind from all the noise. Take deep, relaxing breaths, and by all means, enlist the help of your spouse, family, or friends. While they are watching the baby, take a quick shower and think quiet thoughts. Go for a walk around your block. Sit in your car and listen to your favorite CD, or simply listen to the silence. Then you will be rejuvenated and able to continue to provide comfort to your baby.

Sleepy Baby

Breastfed babies, in the early weeks, should not sleep longer than a three-hour period. While a sleepy baby may be good for you to get more rest, your baby is not going to get the nutrients he needs for growth and brain development. Your baby should be fed, at the very least, every two to three hours.

Breastfeeding Management Concerns

Restrictive Feeding Schedule

You should be feeding your breastfed baby on demand, or as often as he wants. By trying to implement a feeding schedule, you can cause your baby to not adequately gain weight and become frustrated with breastfeeding. It can also cause engorgement if you're only feeding every four hours, for example. Get used to the notion that your role in the beginning is to be there for your baby, providing for his nutritional and emotional needs.

Questionable Milk Supply

Many women become concerned about their milk supply. This is because we can't see how much milk we're making, or how much the baby is actually consuming. You can be sure that you have a sufficient milk supply if your baby looks healthy, is gaining weight, and is producing the necessary number of wet/soiled diapers. To increase your milk supply, allow your baby to breastfeed frequently, both during the day and over the night. Make sure that your baby is emptying both breasts at each feeding. Pump your milk between feedings and store the milk in your freezer. Don't use supplements, especially before four to six weeks. Don't use a pacifier. Let your baby be pacified at your breasts. Get plenty of rest and exercise, and eat a healthy diet. When you're stressed, your milk supply may suffer. Even if the only way to relax is to read a novel or talk on the phone while breastfeeding, take that time. A more relaxed mother creates more breast milk.

Some women find that using the herb fenugreek is helpful in increasing their milk supply. Fenugreek is generally considered to be safe to take while breastfeeding. Most women find a marked increase in their milk supply by taking three fenugreek capsules, three times a day. However, please read the label to see the recommended dosage.

Contact Your Physician Right Away

Certain situations and/or emotions must be handled by a physician. These are outside the realm of normal breastfeeding conditions. If you experience any of these, please contact your physician immediately.

In the mother:
- ❖ Recent chicken pox or measles exposure
- ❖ History of drug use (recreational)
- ❖ HIV positive
- ❖ Anorexia, bulimia
- ❖ Alcohol abuse
- ❖ Hepatitis B
- ❖ No signs of milk production
- ❖ Unrelieved engorgement
- ❖ Bilateral mastitis
- ❖ Recurrent mastitis
- ❖ Breast abscess
- ❖ Postpartum psychosis

In the baby:
- ❖ **Signs of dehydration.** Dehydration, or inadequate supple of fluids to the body, can occur if a baby has been sick, such as with the flu, has diarrhea and/or vomiting, among other health issues. Babies are

more susceptible to dehydration than older children and adults. If a baby is ill, he may not want to drink, so it's important to know the signs, which include:

❖ Fewer than normal wet diapers in a twenty-four-hour period
❖ Unhealthy-looking skin and general appearance of the baby
❖ Lack of tears in a baby over three months
❖ Flattened fontanel, the soft area on the baby's head
❖ Weight loss
❖ Projectile vomiting
❖ Lethargy
❖ Diarrhea and/or vomiting with refusal to nurse
❖ Frothy/odorous stools
❖ Blood in the stool

❖ **Cleft palate and/or lip, short frenulum.** A cleft lip and palate are both present at birth. It is recognized immediately because the lip looks split, and the palate, the soft area at the roof of your mouth, is split as well. A baby with a cleft lip will have surgery to repair the lip during the first few days of life. For a baby with a cleft palate, surgery will take place between six months and three years. Breastfeeding is especially important for a baby with a cleft lip/palate because it helps with bonding. It also helps prevent ear infections, which babies with cleft palate are more susceptible to. It will be necessary to work closely with a lactation professional to find the best position to make breastfeeding work.

❖ **Neurological impairment.** A neurological impairment may include Down's syndrome, neural-tube defeats (e.g., spinal cord, bowel functions, etc.), and other problems that are often present at birth. Because a baby suffering from a neurological disorder will generally have difficulty with sucking adequately, it is important to work closely with a lactation consultant and/or physician.

❖ **Weight Loss.** Initial loss of more than 10 percent of birth weight, failure to regain birth weight by three weeks, and weight gain less than four ounces per week.

❖ **Premature baby under thirty-four weeks.**

❖ **Any normal nursing issues not responding to optimal lactation management.**

❖ **No weight gain in first weeks.**

WEANING MADE EASY

Weaning should occur when you or your baby are ready. Many babies will wean themselves, especially as they approach nine or ten months. You may decide that you're ready to stop breastfeeding. Breastfeeding takes two. If one party is ready to end the experience, then breastfeeding should stop. People may try to make you feel guilty about being ready to stop breastfeeding, whether you've been nursing for a few months or years. You should stop when you're ready. Hopefully, however, you can breastfeed for at least six months.

It's best to wean your baby gradually. This is important so that: you won't experience painful engorgement, your baby won't experience any anxiety about no longer receiving your milk and bonding, and you can resign yourself to the fact that breastfeeding will end. While many women are ready to end breastfeeding for a number of personal reasons, they still tend to feel a sense of wanting to continue because of that emotional bonding that breastfeeding creates. The morning and bedtime feedings are the most difficult to alleviate, so many

(continued)

women stop all other daytime feedings before tackling them. To wean your baby gradually:

❖ Reduce one feeding every three days or so. For example, begin to eliminate perhaps the noontime feeding. Don't breastfeed at noon for about three days. By the third (give or take a day), your baby will no longer expect to be breastfed at noon. Then you can work on eliminating additional feedings, one at a time.

❖ Be honest with your baby, especially if you're weaning an older baby or toddler. Tell him, "Soon you won't be getting Mommy's milk. You'll get (include whatever you're transitioning to)." Babies, and especially toddlers, understand what you're saying to them; after all, they quickly learn what "no," "don't," and "stop" mean.

❖ Get Dad involved! Let him share in the weaning experience. He can take the baby for a walk, play with him, or do anything that will occupy your baby's time and attention during the feeding you are trying to eliminate.

❖ Offer a replacement for a feeding. If your baby is old enough, offer juice or breast milk from a cup. Read a book or play a game.

❖ When you're working on ending a feeding, get out of the house. Don't be near that favorite nursing chair.

❖ To end the nighttime or morning feeding, you may want to change your routine. Offer a cup or bottle instead of the breast.

Important Facts and Helpful Tips about Common Breastfeeding Concerns from a Leading Breastfeeding Professional, Dr. Jack Newman

Reprinted with permission

You Can Still Breastfeed

Over the years, many, many, many women have been wrongly told to stop breastfeeding. The decision about continuing breastfeeding, when the mother must take a drug, for example, involves more than consideration of whether the medication appears in the mother's milk. It also involves taking into consideration the risks of formula-feeding for the baby, which are substantial, the risks of not breastfeeding for the mother, which are substantial, and other issues as well. For example, feeding a breastfeeding baby by bottle for the time the mother is on medication (rarely less than five days), will very often result in the baby refusing the breast forever, or at least becoming very difficult on the breast. On the other hand, it should be taken into consideration that some babies just will not take bottles, so the advice to stop is not only usually wrong, but impractical as well. Furthermore, it is easy to advise the mother to pump her milk when she is not feeding the baby, but adequate pumping is often very difficult to do for some mothers, with the result that the mothers may become very painfully engorged, which may further lead to serious complications.

Breastfeeding and Maternal Medication

Most drugs appear in the milk, but only in very tiny amounts. Although very few drugs may still cause problems for infants even in tiny doses, this is not the case for the vast majority. Mothers who are told they must stop breastfeeding because of a certain drug should ask to be prescribed an alternative medication that is acceptable for breastfeeding mothers. In this day and age, it is rarely a problem to find such an alternative. If the prescribing physician does not know how to proceed, he/she should get more information. If the prescribing physician is not flexible, the mother should seek another opinion.

Most drugs may be considered safe for the mother to take and continue breastfeeding if:

❖ They are commonly prescribed for infants. Examples are amoxicillin, cloxicillin, and most antibiotics.

❖ They are considered safe in pregnancy. Drugs enter directly into the baby's bloodstream when used during pregnancy. The baby generally gets much higher doses, at a much more sensitive period, during pregnancy than during breastfeeding. This is not an absolute, however, as during pregnancy the mother's liver and kidneys will get rid of the drug for the baby.

❖ They are not absorbed from the stomach or intestines. These include many drugs that are given by injection. Examples are gentamicin, heparin, lidocaine, or other local anesthetics used by dentists.

The following frequently used drugs are also generally safe during breastfeeding:

Acetaminophen (Tylenol, Tempra), alcohol (in reasonable amounts), aspirin (in usual doses, for short periods), most anti-epileptic medications, most antihypertensive medications, tetracycline, codeine, most nonsteroidal anti-inflammatory medications, prednisone, thyroxine, propylthiouracil (PTU), warfarin, tricyclic antidepressant medications, sertraline (Zoloft), paroxetine (Paxil), other antidepressants, metronidazole (Flagyl), Nix, Kwellada. Medications applied to the skin, inhaled, or applied to the eyes or nose are almost always safe for breastfeeding.

You can still breastfeed after general, regional, or local anesthesia, as soon as you are up to it. Medications you might take afterwards for pain are almost always permitted.

Immunizations given to the mother do not require her to stop breast-feeding (including with live viruses such as German measles, hepatitis A and B).

Get reliable information before stopping breastfeeding. Once you have stopped, it may be very difficult to start again, especially if the baby is very young.

Breastfeeding and Maternal Illness

Very few maternal illnesses require the mother to stop breastfeeding. This is particularly true of infections. Most infections are caused by viruses. Most infections caused by viruses are most infectious before the mother realizes she is sick. By the time the mother has a fever (or cold, runny nose, diarrhea, vomiting, rash, etc.), she has already passed on the infection to the baby. However, breastfeeding protects the baby against infection, and the mother should thus continue breastfeeding in order to protect the baby. If the baby does get sick, he usually is less sick than if breastfeeding had stopped. But often breastfeeding mothers are pleasantly surprised that their babies do not get sick at all. The baby was protected by his mother's milk.

The only exception to the above is HIV infection in the mother. Until we have more information, it is considered safer for the baby that the mother who is HIV positive not breastfeed, at least when the risks of bottle-feeding are acceptable. There are situations, however, where the risk of not breastfeeding is elevated enough that the mother who is HIV positive should nevertheless breastfeed her baby. The final word is not in, however.

Most other maternal illnesses raise questions because of the drugs the mother might have to take. These should rarely be a problem (see above).

X-rays and Scans

Ordinary X-rays do not require a mother to stop breastfeeding, even when used with contrast (e.g., IVP). CT and MRI scans, even when used with contrast, do not require a mother to stop. A radioactive scan (e.g., lung scan, bone scan) does not require a mother to stop. The only exception is a thyroid scan. However, most of the time the thyroid scan does not have to be done.

A not-uncommon problem in the early months after delivery is a condition called postpartum thyroiditis, a temporary derangement in the thyroid gland's function. A useful test to help understand the condition is a thyroid scan. However, the test requires that radioactive iodine be given to the mother, and this material must not be given to nursing mothers. The radioactive iodine will be found in the milk for weeks, and concentrated in the baby's thyroid. There are ways of dealing with postpartum thyroiditis without doing this test. The drugs a mother might have to take to treat postpartum thyroiditis are compatible with continued breastfeeding (e.g., propranolol, propylthiouracil).

Breast Problems

Mastitis (breast infection) and breast abscess are not reasons to stop breastfeeding. Although surgery on a lactating breast is more difficult, the surgery does not necessarily become easier if the mother stops breastfeeding, as milk continues to be formed for weeks after stopping breastfeeding.

Mammograms are more difficult to read if the mother is breastfeeding, but can still be useful. Once again, how long must a mother wait for her breast to no longer be considered lactating? Evaluation of a lump can be done by other means besides mammography. Discuss options with your doctor. Let him/her know breastfeeding is important to you. A needle biopsy, for example, can be done if a lump is of concern.

New Pregnancy

There is no reason that you cannot continue breastfeeding if you become pregnant. There is no evidence that this does any harm to you, to the baby in your womb, or to the one who is nursing. If you wish to stop breastfeeding, take your time and wean slowly.

Infant Problems

Breastfeeding rarely needs to be discontinued for infant illness. Through breastfeeding, the mother is able to comfort the sick child, and at the same time, the child is able to comfort the mother.

Diarrhea and vomiting

Intestinal infections are rare in exclusively breastfed babies. (Though loose bowel movements are very common). The best treatment for this condition is to continue breastfeeding. The baby will get better more quickly on breast milk. The baby will do well with only breast milk in the vast majority of situations, and will not require added fluids, except in extraordinary cases.

Respiratory illnesses

There is a medical myth that milk should not be given to children with respiratory infections. Whether this is true or not for milk, it is definitely not true for breast milk (and breastfeeding).

Jaundice

Exclusively breastfed babies are commonly jaundiced, even until the third month, though generally the yellow color of the skin is hardly noticeable. Rather than being a problem, this is normal. (There are causes of jaundice that are not normal, but these do not require stopping breastfeeding). If breastfeeding is going well, jaundice does not require the baby to stop breastfeeding. If breastfeeding is not going well, fixing the breastfeeding will improve the jaundice, whereas stopping even for a short time may completely destroy the breastfeeding. Stopping breastfeeding is not the answer.

If the question you have is not discussed above, do not assume that you must stop breastfeeding. Do not stop—get more information. Mothers have been told they must stop breastfeeding for reasons too inane to discuss.

Is My Baby Getting Enough Milk?

Breastfeeding mothers frequently ask how to know their babies are getting enough milk. The breast is not the bottle, and it is not possible to hold the breast up to the light to see how many ounces of milk the baby drank. Our numbers-obsessed society makes it difficult for some mothers to accept not seeing exactly how much milk the baby receives. However, there are ways of knowing that the baby is getting enough. In the long run, weight gain is the best indication of whether the baby is getting enough, but rules about weight gain appropriate for bottle-fed babies may not be appropriate for breastfed babies.

Ways of Knowing
1. Baby's nursing is characteristic.

A baby who is obtaining good amounts of milk at the breast sucks in a very characteristic way. When a baby is getting milk (he is not getting milk just because he has the breast in his mouth and is making sucking movements), you will see a pause at the point of his chin after he opens to the maximum and before he closes his mouth (open mouth wide→pause→close mouth). If you wish to demonstrate this to yourself, put your finger in your mouth and suck as if you were sucking on a straw. As you draw in, your chin drops and stays down as long as you are drawing in. When you stop drawing in, your chin comes back up. This pause that is visible at the baby's chin represents a mouthful of milk when the baby does it at the breast. The longer the pause, the more the baby got. Once you know about the pause you can cut through so much of the nonsense breastfeeding mothers are being told—like feed the baby twenty minutes on each side. A baby who does this type of sucking (with the pauses) for twenty 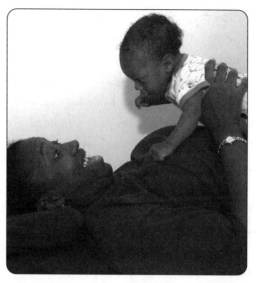 minutes straight might not even take the second side. A baby who nibbles (doesn't drink) for twenty hours will come off the breast hungry.

2. Swallowing.

When your baby has a good latch and is nursing efficiently, you should be able to hear him swallow. It may sound like gulping, too, but it's characteristic swallowing of your breast milk that you hear. Please remember to burp your baby after each feeding, even between switching breasts, as air can still get in and gas may occur. Rubbing or gently patting your baby's back is generally effective. Beware, however, that hearing your baby burp may take some time. You might notice that your baby spits up after feeding. This is normal. Some babies spit up rarely, while others seem to do so frequently.

3. Baby's bowel movements.

For the first few days after delivery, the baby passes meconium, a dark green, almost black, substance. Meconium accumulates in the baby's gut during pregnancy. Meconium is passed during the first few days, and by the third day, the bowel movements start becoming lighter as more breast milk is taken. Usually by the fifth day, the bowel movements have taken on the appearance of the normal breast milk stool. The normal breast milk stool is pasty to watery, mustard colored, and usually has little odor. However, bowel movements may vary considerably from this description. They may be green or orange, may contain curds or mucus, or may resemble shaving cream in consistency (from air bubbles). The variation in color does not mean something is wrong. A baby who is breastfeeding only and is starting to have bowel movements that are becoming lighter by day three of life is doing well.

Without your becoming obsessive about it, monitoring the frequency and quantity of bowel motions is one of the best ways of knowing if the baby is getting enough milk (but not as good as observing the pause in the chin). After the first three to four days, the baby should have increasing bowel movements so that, by the end of the first week, he should be passing at least two to three substantial yellow stools each day. In addition, many infants have a stained diaper with almost each feeding. A baby who is still passing meconium on the fourth or fifth day of life should be seen by a doctor the same day. A baby who is passing only brown bowel movements is probably not getting enough, but this is not a very reliable indicator.

After the first three to four weeks of life, some breastfed babies may suddenly change their stool pattern from many each day to one every three days, or even less. Some babies have gone as long as fifteen days or more without a bowel movement. As long as the baby is otherwise well, and the stool is the usual pasty or soft, yellow movement, this is not constipation and is of no concern. No treatment is necessary or desirable, because no treatment is necessary or desirable for something that is normal.

Any baby between five and twenty-one days of age who does not pass at least one substantial bowel movement within a twenty-four-hour period should be seen by a pediatrician the same day. Generally, small, infrequent bowel movements during this time period mean insufficient intake. There are definitely some exceptions and everything may be fine, but it is better to check.

4. Urination.

With six soaking wet (not just wet) diapers in a twenty-four-hour period, after about four to five days of life, you can be sure that the baby is getting a lot of milk (if he is only breastfeeding). Unfortunately, the new super-dry "disposable" diapers often do indeed feel dry even when full of urine, but when soaked with urine they are heavy. It should be obvious that this indication of milk intake does not apply if you are giving the baby extra water (which, in any case, is unnecessary for breastfed babies, and if given by bottle, may interfere with breastfeeding). The baby's urine should be almost colorless after the first few days, though an occasional darker urine is not of concern.

During the first two to three days of life, some babies pass pink or red urine. This is not a reason to panic, and does not mean the baby is dehydrated. No one knows what it means, or even if it is abnormal. It is undoubtedly associated with the lesser intake of the breastfed baby, compared with the bottle-fed baby during this time, but the bottle-feeding baby is not the standard on which to judge breastfeeding. However, the appearance of this color urine should result in attention to getting the baby well latched on, and making sure the baby is drinking at the breast. During the first few days of life, only if the baby is well latched on can he get his mother's milk. Giving water by bottle or cup or finger-feeding at this point does not fix the problem. Fixing the latch usually fixes the problem. If relatching and breast compression do not result in better intake, there are ways of giving extra fluid without giving a bottle directly. Limiting the duration or frequency of feedings can also contribute to a decreased intake of milk.

The Following are Not Good Ways of Judging
1. Your breasts do not feel full.

After the first few days or weeks, it is usual for most mothers not to feel full. Your body adjusts to your baby's requirements. This change may occur quite suddenly. Some mothers who breastfeed perfectly well never feel engorged or full.

2. The baby sleeps through the night.

A baby who is sleeping through the night at ten days of age, for example, may, in fact, not be getting enough milk. A baby who is too sleepy and has to be awakened for feeds, or who is "too good" may not be getting enough milk. There are many exceptions, but get help quickly.

3. The baby cries after feeding.

Although the baby may cry after feeding because of hunger, there are also many other reasons for crying. This is referring to a baby that still cries, even after being breastfed. The key is to let the baby nurse till full, without rushing through or limiting a feeding. Then offer the other breast, after the first one is empty, to ensure that the baby gets enough milk.

4. The baby feeds often and/or for a long time.

For one mother, feedings every three hours or so may be often; for another, three hours or so may be a long period between feeds. For one, a feeding that lasts for thirty minutes is a long feeding; for another, it is a short one. There are no rules how often or for how long a baby should nurse. It is not true that the baby gets 90 percent of the feed in the first ten minutes. Let the baby determine his own feeding schedule and things usually work right, if the baby is suckling and drinking at the breast, and having at least two to three substantial yellow bowel movements each day. Remember, a baby may be on the breast for two hours, but if he is actually feeding (open wide→pause→close mouth type of sucking) for only two minutes, he will come off the breast hungry. If the baby falls asleep quickly at the breast, you can compress the breast to continue the flow of milk. Contact your physician or breastfeeding professional with any concerns, but wait to start supplementing. If supplementation is truly necessary, there are ways of supplementing that do not use an artificial nipple.

5. "I can express only half an ounce of milk."

This means nothing and should not influence you. Therefore, you should not pump your breasts "just to know." Most mothers have plenty of milk. The problem usually is that the baby is not getting the milk that is available, either because he is latched on poorly, or the suckle is ineffective, or both. These problems can often be fixed easily.

6. The baby will take a bottle after feeding.

This does not necessarily mean that the baby is still hungry. This is not a good test, as bottles may interfere with breastfeeding. The five-week-old is suddenly pulling away from the breast, but still seems hungry. This does not mean your milk has "dried up" or decreased. During the first few weeks of life, babies often fall asleep at the breast when the flow of milk slows down, even if they have not had their fill. When they are older (four to six weeks of age), they no longer are content to fall asleep, but rather start to pull away or get upset. The milk supply has not changed; the baby has. Compress the breast to increase flow.

Protocol to Increase Intake of Breast Milk by the Baby

Here is the way I suggest mothers proceed for "insufficient milk supply" (actually, most mothers have lots, but the problem is that the baby is not getting the milk that is available).

1. Get the best latch possible. This needs to be shown by someone who knows what they are doing. Anyone can look at a baby at the breast and say the latch is good. If a mother has plenty of milk, the latch does not have to be perfect. But if the milk supply is decreased, the baby will get more milk if he is latched on better. Get good "hands-on" help.

2. Once the baby is no longer drinking on his own, use compression to increase flow to the baby. Compression can be particularly helpful, but don't forget trying to get the best latch possible first. Babies tend to pull at the breast when the flow of milk is slow, so it is useful to know how to know the baby is actually getting milk and not just sucking without getting milk. When the baby no longer seems to be getting milk, or is sucking without getting milk, this is when to start compression. Keep the baby on the first breast until he doesn't drink even with compression.

3. When the baby no longer drinks, even with compression, switch sides and repeat the process. Keep going back and forth as long as the baby gets reasonable amounts of milk at the breast.

4. Try fenugreek and blessed thistle. These two herbs seem to increase milk supply and the rate of milk flow.

In the evening, when babies often want to be at the breast for long periods, get help to position the baby so that you can feed lying down. Let the baby nurse, and maybe you will fall asleep. Or rent videos and let the baby nurse while you watch.

It is not always easy to decide if a baby needs supplementation. Sometimes more rapid growth is necessary, and it may not be possible without supplementation. If possible, get banked breast milk to use as a

NOTES ON SCALES AND WEIGHTS

Scales are all different. We have documented significant differences from one scale to another. Weights have often been written down wrong. A soaked cloth diaper may weigh 250 grams (half a pound) or more, so babies should be weighed naked or with a brand new dry diaper. Many rules about weight gain are taken from observations of growth of formula-feeding babies. They do not necessarily apply to breastfeeding babies. A slow start may be compensated for later, by adjusting the breastfeeding. Growth charts are guidelines only.

supplement. If not available, formula may be necessary. However, sometimes slow but steady growth is acceptable. The main reason to worry about growth is that good growth is one sign of good health. A baby who grows well is usually in good health, but this is not necessarily so. Neither is a baby who grows slowly in poor health, but physicians worry about a baby who is growing more slowly than average. Growth charts are frequently interpreted poorly. A baby who follows the tenth percentile line is growing as he should be. Too many people, including physicians, believe that only babies on the fiftieth percentile or higher are growing normally. Not true. Growth charts were developed on information gathered about normal babies. Somebody has got to be smaller than 90 percent of all other babies. Somebody normal.

If it is decided to supplement, the best way is at the breast with a lactation aid. Introduce the supplement with a nursing supplementer (lactation aid), not a bottle, syringe, cup, or finger-feeding. Supplement only after steps three and four, and the baby has nursed on at least both sides. A baby learns to breastfeed by breastfeeding, and there is more to breastfeeding than the breast milk. Keep the baby at the breast! Why is it better to use the lactation aid?

❖ Babies learn to breastfeed by breastfeeding.

❖ Mothers learn to breastfeed by breastfeeding.

❖ The baby continues to get your milk.

❖ The baby won't reject the breast.

❖ There is more to breastfeeding than the breast milk.

If the baby is older than three or four months and supplementation appears to be necessary, formula is *not* necessary, and extra calories can be given to the baby as solid foods. First solids may include: mashed banana, mashed avocado, mashed potato or sweet potato, and infant cereals, as much as the baby will take and after the baby has nursed, if he is still hungry. Even at this age, giving bottles when the baby is not getting much from the breast will often result in breast rejection. If you must give formula, mix it with the solids. Giving solids at three or four months is not recommended if everything is going well, and even if the weight gain is slow, there are several ways of getting the baby more breast milk that can be tried before adding solids. Solids should normally be started when the baby is showing interest in eating solids (usually around five or six months of age).

Starting Solid Foods

Breast milk is all your baby needs until at least four months of age. Most babies will do fine with exclusive breastfeeding until six months of age or longer. Why start solid foods?

❖ Because there comes a time when breast milk no longer supplies all your baby's nutritional needs. (This does not mean, as some uninformed people say, that there is no nutritional value in breast milk after the baby is six months old). A full-term baby will start requiring iron from other sources by six to nine months of age. The calories supplied by breast milk may become inadequate by eight to nine months of age, although some babies can continue to grow well on breast milk alone well past a year.

❖ Because some babies who are not started on solids by a certain age (nine to twelve months) may have great difficulty accepting solid foods.

❖ Because it is a developmental milestone that your child passes when he starts solid foods. He is growing up. Usually, he will want to eat solids. Why stop him?

When to Start Solid Foods

The best time to start solids is when the baby is showing interest in starting. Some babies will become very interested in the food on their parents' plates as early as four months of age. By five or six months of age, most babies will be reaching for and trying to grab food that parents have on their plates. When the baby is starting to reach for food, this seems a reasonable time to start giving him some. There really is no reason to start on a specific date. Go by the baby's cues.

In some cases, it may be better to start food earlier. When a baby seems to be hungry, or when weight gain is not continuing at the desired rate, it may be reasonable to start solids as early as three months of age. Starting at three months of age when things are going well, however, is not recommended (see above). However, it may be possible, with help, to continue breastfeeding alone and have the baby less hungry and/or growing more rapidly. There is no advantage to giving artificial baby milk (formula) and there may be some disadvantages. The baby who is not satisfied completely at the breast may start to take more and more from the bottle, and end up refusing to take the breast.

The breastfed baby digests solid foods better and earlier than the formula-fed baby because breast milk contains enzymes that help digest fats, proteins, and starch. Also, breastfed babies have had a wide variety of tastes in their lives, since the flavors of many foods the mother eats will pass into her milk. Breastfed babies thus accept solids more readily than artificially fed babies. Breast milk is amazing stuff, eh?

How should solids be introduced?

When the baby is starting to take solids at about five or six months of age, there is little difference what he starts with, or in what order foods are introduced. It is prudent to avoid highly spiced or highly allergenic foods at first (e.g., egg whites, strawberries), but if the baby reaches for the potato on your plate, make sure it is not too hot, and let him have the potato. There is no need to go in any specific order, and there is no need for the baby to eat only one food for a certain period of time. Some exclusively breastfed babies dislike infant cereal when it is introduced at five or six months of age. There is no need for concern and no need to persist if the baby doesn't want the cereal. There is nothing magic or necessary about infant cereal. Offer your baby the foods that he is interested in. Allow the baby to enjoy food, and do not worry exactly how much he actually takes at first. Much of it may end up in his hair and on the floor anyhow. There is no need, either, that foods be pureed if the baby is five or six months of age or older. Simple mashing with a fork is all that is necessary at first. You also do not have to be exceedingly careful about how much the baby takes. Why limit the baby to one teaspoon if he wants more? You do not need to waste your money on commercial baby foods.

Be relaxed, feed the baby at your mealtimes, and as he becomes a more accomplished eater of solid foods, offer a greater variety of foods at any one time:

❖ The easiest way to get extra iron for your baby of five or six months of age is by giving him meat. Infant cereal has iron, but it is poorly absorbed and may cause the baby to be constipated.

❖ There is no reason to introduce vegetables before fruit. Breast milk is far sweeter than fruit, so there is no reason to believe that the baby will take vegetables better by delaying the introduction of fruit.

❖ Respect your baby's likes and dislikes. There is no essential food (except breast milk). If your baby does not like a certain food, do not push it on him. If you think it important for him, wait a few weeks and offer it again.

At about eight months of age, babies become somewhat assertive in displaying their individuality. Your baby may not want you to put a spoon into his mouth. He very likely will take it out of your hand and put it into his mouth himself, often upside down, so that the food falls on his lap. Respect his attempts at self-sufficiency and encourage his learning.

What if I am starting solids at three months?

At this age, it may be prudent to go a little more slowly. Start with infant cereal or easily mashed foods, such as bananas. Sometimes a baby will eat better from your fingers than off a spoon. Go a little more slowly with quantities as well. As the baby tolerates solids, both quantity and variety of foods can be increased, as the baby desires.

Solids or breast first?

There seems to be considerable worry when a child is starting solids about whether to give the breast or solid food first. If breastfeeding and the introduction of solid foods both are going well, it probably does not matter much. Indeed, there is no reason that a baby needs both breast and solids every time he eats.

Chapter Four

We Shall Overcome
Breastfeeding Barriers

Breastfeeding barriers are those issues, experiences, and beliefs women embrace, that interfere with their breastfeeding success. Barriers are challenges that get in the way of your breastfeeding experience. They may be related to your environment, the people around you, society, cultural traditions, world events, or economics. Barriers may also be rooted deeply in fear, inner beliefs, abuse, self-esteem, or other interpersonal issues. Barriers are based on identifiable facts and/or unlikely possibilities—whatever you believe to be a barrier *is* a barrier to you.

The question is: How will you overcome that barrier? For instance, a woman may not be able to afford the purchase of a breast pump. So, she may decide to stop breastfeeding once she returns to work. The fact is that she does not have the money to buy a breast pump. What can she do? Another example of a barrier based on fact is that a woman may feel pressure to stop breastfeeding after a year. The fact is that it's not the "normal" practice for women to breastfeed in this country past their child's first birthday. What can she do? One woman may be hesitant about breastfeeding because she was sexually abused, and can't even visualize her baby attached to her breasts. What are her options? Another woman may believe that breast milk will not be sufficient to nourish her baby. What will she do?

Breastfeeding barriers are as diverse and individual as African American women. The benefit of being an African American woman who has to face a breastfeeding barrier is that we have an intense cultural legacy of overcoming massive struggle in the areas of slavery, racism, prejudice, sexism, and inequality in the workplace, among other things. If we as a race of women can survive those life atrocities, then we can surely overcome breastfeeding barriers.

Barrier: Culture

Today, the African American culture is not largely focused on breastfeeding. Since we have not breastfed for generations, we don't have that family link to this tradition. We rarely have breastfeeding role models in our community who are examples of how breastfeeding works. Many of us will be the first mothers in generations in our families to resume the lost art of breastfeeding. This barrier can be tricky to overcome because it means making a stand in uncharted waters. Breastfeeding is not a normal occurrence in our community anymore, so you'll be blazing trails that will have a positive impact on your street, in your neighborhood, within your family, and in the greater Black community for many years to come.

What You Can Do

❖ **Take a stand!** By breastfeeding your baby, you already know the emotional and physical benefits for both of you. You'll change the course of your baby's life and increase his chances for healthy living in the future. Even further than that, your decision to breastfeed will be the motivation for others around you to breastfeed their own babies. You'll be a role model to your friends, family, and other women around you. You'll be making a statement that says, "I care about my baby enough to do the best for him, regardless of how anyone feels about it." Women will notice, and start to ask you questions about breastfeeding. Your commitment to provide the best for your baby will change our generational absence of breastfeeding to one that will ensure a healthier African American community.

❖ **Educate yourself!** Read as much as you can about breastfeeding and how it benefits you, your baby, and society as a whole. Learn about the many health problems that plague our Black babies, and how the simple act of breastfeeding can greatly prevent and reduce these illnesses, including asthma, childhood diabetes, and obesity. Do your own research about lactose intolerance in our community and how breastfeeding can protect your baby from developing it. Go online and read studies on how breastfeeding can reduce the high rate of infant mortality in our community. Remember: knowledge is power.

Barrier: Myths

One of the major barriers to breastfeeding in our community is a widespread belief in breastfeeding myths. *Breast milk is not enough to feed a baby. Breastfeeding is painful. My milk will dry up. I'll be tied down with the baby.* These myths, like any myth on any topic, tend to be a mixture of distorted facts and miseducation.

What You Can Do

❖ **Learn the myths about breastfeeding.** Discover the truths to address those myths.

❖ **Stand your ground.** People will believe what they want to believe. The facts can be presented in clear language, but some people will refuse to see the truth. It's easier for some people to live in denial, than to have to face reality. When this happens, share what you know and keep moving. Don't weaken because someone doesn't believe your factual information. They may need more time to think about what you've shared. They may come around later, but feel confident that you've done your part by presenting the truth.

Barrier: Lack of Education and Support

Another significant barrier in our community is a lack of breastfeeding education and support. Health care providers have long neglected pregnant African American women in this area of prenatal care. Few Black women receive breastfeeding education during the prenatal period. If they do, it tends to be outside of their health care provider or community. Doctors, on a large scale, do not educate us about breastfeeding. It's a widespread assumption that, since most Black women don't breastfeed, there's no reason to share breastfeeding information. Ironically, obstetricians and pediatricians rarely receive breastfeeding education during medical school. So, they are often not even qualified to share an in-depth knowledge of the advantages of breastfeeding, and how it works. Black women on the WIC program tend to receive more breastfeeding education than women who aren't on the program, but even then it depends on how breastfeeding-friendly each individual WIC agency is.

Just as we receive insufficient breastfeeding education during pregnancy, there are even fewer places to receive support once we decide to breastfeed. A very small number of African American communities have breastfeeding support groups. Women who seek support will have to venture outside of their community. Black women sometimes find that they are the only Black in the support group. This may be uncomfortable for her and the other women in the group. Many Black women only attend a few meetings outside of their communities before giving up, saying, "I didn't feel comfortable" or "their views on parenting were different" or "they wanted to force their parenting lifestyle on everyone in the group."

Also, these groups don't always cater to our needs. Since many of us work, it's nearly impossible for us to attend a breastfeeding support group that meets at ten o'clock on Wednesday mornings.

In addition, husbands, boyfriends, girlfriends, and other family members may not support our decision to breastfeed because it's no longer a normal part of the African American experience, they believe breastfeeding myths, or they don't have good information about breastfeeding.

What You Can Do

❖ **Hold your health-care provider accountable.** If you're pregnant and you haven't received any information about breastfeeding, bring it up to your doctor. Ask about his/her beliefs on the importance of breastfeeding, and where you can go for support. You can also ask to be connected with other patients who have breastfed. Discuss any medication you may be taking during pregnancy and if it's safe to take while breastfeeding. Any questions you have about breastfeeding, pose them to your health care provider, which may compel him/her to become more informed. Encourage your doctor to go online to the American Academy of Pediatrics (AAP) www.aap.org. Here, he/she will find a helpful document called "Ten Steps to Support Parents' Choice to Breastfeed Their Baby." Often doctors will be more receptive reading information from their own peers.

❖ **Seek help.** We tend to believe that we can figure problems out and that we can be superwomen. We don't have to be! Believe me, being superwoman is overrated and underpaid! Look for any breastfeeding support groups in your area or a nearby community. Attend the meeting. If you don't feel comfortable, find another one. Ask a friend who breastfed for help. Talk to your WIC agency for breastfeeding resources. Ask your hospital if they have a lactation consultant on duty. If you can't find a group in your area, or if you aren't at ease in the group you find, try another route. Seek out mother support groups or parenting groups that may meet at your local hospital, church, library, or college. Make a phone call to a breastfeeding hotline. Call the African American Breastfeeding Alliance (AABA) at (877) 532-8535. See additional resources at the end of the book.

❖ **Educate yourself and your family.** Again, breastfeeding knowledge equals a better chance at breastfeeding success. Go online, head to the library, or get information from your health care provider on breastfeeding benefits and breastfeeding management.

❖ **Start your own support group.** If you can't find the support you want, start a group to help other mothers. Call a group of pregnant, breastfeeding, or breastfeeding-experienced women together. Meet regularly, and gain confidence and motivation from each other. You'll find that by helping other women with breastfeeding, you feel empowered and gain the inspiration to make it through your own breastfeeding challenges. If you see other Black women who are pregnant, ask them if they're going to breastfeed. This can open a dialogue that may lead to another breastfeeding woman in your community. If you see a Black woman who is breastfeeding in public, go and quietly tell her she's doing a great job. By working together, we can support each other toward breastfeeding success and foster a community of loving, sisterly support. See the resources chapter for more information on starting a group of your own.

Barrier: Inner Doubts

Sometimes our own fears and inner doubts hinder our potential breastfeeding success. Your fears may include: shyness about breastfeeding in public, doing something different than the other mothers in your environment, inability to do it right, a belief that you will lose your sense of freedom if you breastfeed, or the unknown about breastfeeding. You may be concerned about being that close with someone other than your mate. You may have low self-esteem and feel that you just don't have what it takes to breastfeed your baby. Previous sexual abuse may have deeply wounded your ability to even imagine giving that type of love to another person; the thought of having a baby latched on to your breast is unimaginable. Perhaps your breasts are very small or very large, one is larger than the other, your nipples are either flat or inverted. You may assume that you are inadequate or too abundant to provide for your baby.

What You Can Do

❖ **Believe in yourself!** You have what it takes to breastfeed your baby. Your determination to breastfeed is 90 percent of the battle. The rest is education and practice, practice, practice.

❖ **If you've been abused, know that it was not your fault!** You were the victim. Seek support from a professional who can help you through the process of mending the emotional and mental trauma caused by the abuse. Breastfeeding can actually be a part of your emotional healing. By nursing your baby, you can begin to feel deep, personal satisfaction in your own self-worth and in your divine importance as a mother. Just take it one feeding and one day at a time.

❖ **Give thanks for your breasts!** Regardless of the size, shape, or appearance of your breasts, rest assured that they are fully prepared and ready for breastfeeding. If you have experienced breast surgery, including reduction or augmentation, you should check with your physician and surgeon to find out where the incision(s) was made. If your milk ducts and sinuses were not disturbed during your procedure, then it is likely that you can be successful at breastfeeding. If your milk ducts or sinuses were damaged, then you may not be able to breastfeed. If you had surgery on one breast only, and your ducts/sinuses were damaged, then you should be able to breastfeed with the other breast. You may, however, need to supplement with infant formula. You should work closely with a lactation consultant if this is the case. In the event that you're reading this book in preparation for your childbearing years (way to go!) and breast surgery is possible, please inform your physician and surgeon that you plan to breastfeed in the future. Keep a dialogue going, and share this information with them so they can be sure to conduct a surgery that will not hinder breastfeeding success. You were born with all that your baby needs for survival for up to six months of his life. Your breasts are remarkably suited for your baby. Besides, your infant will not care if your breasts are small, large, lopsided, one-sided, or scarred. Your baby will happily receive your life-giving milk unconditionally.

Barrier: Infant Formula

From your first prenatal appointment to the delivery of your baby, you are undoubtedly bombarded with infant formula advertisements. These ads are in many forms: the cool diaper bag you receive at your first prenatal visit that is stocked full of infant formula items, baby magazines full of formula ads, coupons for infant formula, samples of infant formula, videos about pregnancy that are full of formula ads, classical music CDs stamped with infant formula logos, emails with information on how your baby is grow-ing, and literature in clinic or physician waiting rooms on (what else?) infant formula. Infant formula is a two-billion-dollar-a-year industry. The mass marketing of infant formula and formula products, including prepared baby food and vitamin supplements, has been effective in creating the myth that infant formula is just as good as breast milk. Formula companies can afford to market their product in a way that has many of us believing that our babies will get the same benefits from their product as they will from breast milk. These ads make you think that they have your baby's health and your best interest in mind. In spite of decades of research, no formula has come close to replicating the components of breast milk. These companies want you to buy their product, and they will do anything—from multimillion-dollar marketing campaigns to giveaways—to make you their consumer, when they know that you already have what you need for your baby.

What You Can Do

- ❖ **Don't be fooled!** Throw away infant formula marketing materials, like magazines, coupons, and gifts. Do not bring formula into your home. It's too tempting when the going gets rough to reach for the formula instead of the breast!
- ❖ **Be aware.** Infant formula is a substandard substitute for breast milk that does not protect your baby from any illness or disease or sudden infant death syndrome, does not increase your baby's IQ, will not help you lose weight or prevent ovarian and breast cancer, and will cost you at least a thousand dollars—or more—a year to feed one baby. WIC does not provide all the infant formula a baby needs.
- ❖ **Choose wisely.** Commit to breastfeeding your baby. Anyone can feed your baby infant formula, but only you can breastfeed your baby.

Thirteen Risks of Formula-Feeding by INFACT Canada

Adapted from the INFACT Canada's Fourteen Risks Fact Sheet. Reprinted with permission.

When breastfeeding is not fully practiced, infant formulas are generally used. The World Health Organization International Code of Marketing of Breast Milk Substitutes requires that parents be informed about the health hazards of unnecessary or improper use of infant formula. This brief annotated bibliography gives some examples from the extensive body of research documenting the importance of breastfeeding, and in turn the associated risks of formula-feeding. The World Health Organization recommends exclusive breastfeeding for six months, the introduction of nutritious, complementary foods at six months, and continued breastfeeding for two years and beyond.

1. Increased Risk of Asthma

A study of 2,184 children, done by the Hospital for Sick Children in Toronto, determined that the risk of asthma and wheezing was approximately 50 percent higher when infants were formula-fed compared to infants who were breastfed for nine months or longer.

Researchers in West Australia studied 2,602 children to determine the development of asthma and wheeze at six years of age. Not breastfeeding increased the risk of asthma and wheeze by 40 percent, compared to infants who were exclusively breastfed for four months. The authors recommend exclusive breastfeeding for at least four months to reduce the risk of asthma.

The reviewers looked at twenty-nine studies to evaluate the protective effect of breastfeeding against asthma. After applying strict criteria for assessment, fifteen studies remained in the review. All fifteen showed a protective effect of breastfeeding (a risk of formula-feeding). They concluded that the evidence is clear and consistent that breastfeeding protects against asthma.

2. Increased Risk of Allergy

Children in Finland who had been breastfed the longest had the lowest incidence of eczema, food allergies, and respiratory allergies. At seventeen years of age, the incidence of respiratory allergies for those who had little breastfeeding was 65 percent, and for those who were breastfed the longest, 42 percent.

A longitudinal perspective study of 1,246 healthy infants in Arizona aimed to determine the relationship between breastfeeding and recurrent wheezing. The results showed that Nona topic children at the age of six who had not been breastfed were three times more likely to have recurrent wheezing. Infants with a maternal history of respiratory allergies or asthma were assessed for atopic dermatitis during the first year of life. Seventy-six Dutch children with and 228 children without atopic dermatitis were examined. Exclusive breastfeeding for the first three months was found to have a protective effect against dermatitis.

3. Reduced Cognitive Development

A total of 3,880 Australian children were followed from birth to determine breastfeeding patterns, and later, cognitive development. Those breastfed for six months or more scored 8.2 points higher for females, and 5.8 points higher for males in vocabulary tests over those who had never been breastfed.

School-aged children (439), who weighed less than approximately 3.3 pounds at birth, and were born in the U.S. between 1991 and 1993 were given a variety of cognitive tests. The very low-birth-weight infants who were never breastfed were found to have lower test scores in overall intellectual function, verbal ability, visual-spatial, and visual motor skills than those who were breastfed.

To determine the impact of exclusive breastfeeding on cognitive development for infants born small for gestational age, this U.S.-based study evaluated 220 infants, using the Bayley Scales of Infant Development at thirteen months, and the Weschler Preschool and Primary Scales of Intelligence at five years. The researchers concluded that exclusively breast-fed (without supplements), small for gestational age infants had a significant advantage in cognitive development without compromising growth. The benefits of breastfeeding have long-term potential on a person's life through its influence on childhood cognitive and educational development, the study concluded. Regression analysis was used to determine that breast-feeding was significantly and positively associated with educational levels obtained by age twenty-six as well as cognitive abilities at age fifty-three.

4. Increased Risk of Acute Respiratory Disease

A number of sources were used to examine the relationship between breast-feeding and the risk of hospitalization for lower respiratory tract disease in healthy full-term infants with access to adequate health facilities. Analysis of the data concluded that in developed countries, infants who were formula-fed experienced more than three times the severity of respiratory tract illness and required hospitalization, compared to infants who were exclusively breastfed for four months. To determine the modifiable risk factors for acute lower respiratory infection in young children, an Indian hospital–based study compared 201 cases to 311 controls. Lack of breast-feeding was one of the key modifiable risk factors for lower respiratory infection in children under five years of age.

5. Increased Risk of Childhood Cancers

Not breastfeeding is known to increase the risk of cancer. This novel study found a significant level of genetic damage in infants aged nine to twelve months who were not breastfed. The authors speculate that this may play a role in the development of cancer in childhood or later in life. The UK

Childhood Cancer Study analyzed thirty-five hundred childhood cancer cases and the relationship to breastfeeding. Results showed a small reduction for leukemia and for all cancers combined when infants had "ever been breastfed." A case-controlled study in the United Arab Emirates looked at 117 cases of acute lymphocytic leukemia and 117 controls. They found that the breastfeeding duration of those with leukemia was significantly shorter than the breastfeeding duration of the controls. They concluded that breastfeeding duration of six months or longer may protect against childhood acute leukemia and lymphomas.

6. Increased Risk of Chronic Diseases

A review of infant feeding practices and childhood chronic diseases shows increased risk for type 1 diabetes, celiac disease, some childhood cancers, and inflammatory bowel disease associated with artificial infant feeding. Celiac disease may be triggered by an autoimmune response when an infant is exposed to a food containing gluten proteins. In order to investigate the impact of breastfeeding on this response, Ivarsson and her team of researchers looked at the breastfeeding patterns of 627 children with celiac disease and at 1,254 healthy children to determine the effect of breastfeeding during the time of introduction of gluten-containing foods on the outcome of the development of celiac disease. An astounding 40 percent risk reduction was reported for the development of celiac disease in children at two years of age or younger for those who were breastfed when dietary gluten was introduced. And the effect was even more pronounced in infants who continued to be breastfed after dietary gluten was introduced, the authors noted.

7. Increased Risk of Diabetes

Early introduction of infant formula, solids, and cow's milk are factors shown to increase the incidence of type 1 diabetes later in life. Swedish (517) and Lithuanian (286) children aged zero to fifteen years who were diagnosed with type 1 diabetes were compared to controls. The results showed that exclusive breastfeeding for longer than five months, and total breastfeeding for longer than seven or nine months, is protective against diabetes. To determine the link between cow's milk consumption (cow's milk–based infant formula) and the development of antibody response to cow's milk protein, Italian researchers measured the antibody response of sixteen breastfed and twelve cow's milk–fed infants under four months of age. Cow's milk–fed infants had elevated levels of beta-casein antibodies when compared to breastfed infants. The researchers concluded that breastfeeding for the first four months prevented the production of antibodies and could have a preventive effect on the development of type 1 diabetes. In this case-controlled study, forty-six native Canadian type 2 diabetes patients were matched with ninety-two controls. Prenatal and postnatal risk factors were compared. Breastfeeding was found to reduce the risk of type 2 diabetes.

8. Increased Risk of Cardiovascular Disease

A prospective study followed 7,276 term UK infants for 7.5 years. Full data was available for 4,763 children. For those not breastfed, both systolic and diastolic pressures were found to be higher at age seven than for those who were breastfed.

There was a 0.2 mm mercury reduction for each three months of breast-feeding. The authors suggest there may be significant benefits during adult-hood as a 1 percent reduction in population systolic blood pressure is associated with a 1.5 percent reduction in overall mortality.

This UK study looked at the cholesterol levels of fifteen hundred thirteen- to sixteen-year-olds and determined that breastfeeding may have long-term benefits in preventing cardiovascular disease by reducing the total cholesterol and the low-density lipid cholesterol. The research suggests that early exposure to breast milk may program fat metabolism in later life, resulting in lower blood cholesterol levels, and therefore a lower risk of cardiovascular disease.

To confirm links between infant nutrition and health risks in later life, British researchers measured the blood pressure of 216 children at thirteen to sixteen years of age who had been born prematurely. For those who had received preterm infant formula or routine infant formula, blood pressure was higher than for those who had received breast milk during infancy. The authors concluded that for children born prematurely, breastfeeding lowers blood pressure in later life, and that this conclusion can be extended to term infants as well.

9. Increased Risk of Obesity

In order to determine factors associated with the development of obesity, 6,650 German school-aged children between the ages five and fourteen years of age were examined. Breastfeeding was found to be protective against obesity. The protective effect was greater when the infants were exclusively breastfed. To determine the impact of infant feeding on childhood obesity, this large Scottish study looked at the body mass index of 32,200 children aged thirty-nine to forty-two months. After elimination of confounding factors, socioeconomic status, birth weight, and sex, the prevalence of obesity was significantly higher in the formula-fed children, leading to the conclusion that formula-feeding is associated with an increase in childhood obesity risk.

German researchers collected height and weight data of 9,375 schoolchildren to determine the impact of early childhood feeding on the development of obesity. The prevalence of obesity was found to be 4.5 percent —nearly 40 percent higher—in those who had never been breastfed compared to 2.8 percent for those who had been exclusively breastfed.

10. Increased Risk of Gastrointestinal Infections

A comparison between infants who received primarily breast milk during the first twelve months of life and infants who were exclusively formula-fed or who were breastfed for three months or less found that diarrheal disease was twice as high for the formula-fed infants as for those who were breastfed. Seven hundred and seventy-six infants from New Brunswick, Canada, were assessed for the relationship between respiratory and gastrointestinal illnesses and breastfeeding during the first six months of life. Although the rates of exclusive breastfeeding were low, the results showed breastfeeding had a significant protective effect against total illness during the first six months of life. For those breastfed, the incidence of gastrointestinal infections was 47 percent lower; the rate of respiratory disease was 34 percent lower than for those who were not breastfed. Breastfeeding promotion in Belarus significantly reduced the incidence of gastrointestinal infections by 40 percent.

11. Increased Risk of Mortality

The researchers examined 1,204 infants who died between twenty-eight days and one year of age from causes other than congenital anomaly or malignant tumor, and 7,740 children who were still alive at one year to calculate mortality and whether or not the infant was breastfed as well as the duration-response effects. Children who were never breastfed had a 21 percent greater risk of dying in the postneonatal period than those who were breastfed. Longer breastfeeding was associated with lower risk. Promoting breastfeeding has the potential to prevent about seven hundred twenty postneonatal deaths in the United States each year. In Canada, this would be about seventy-two deaths. Compared with exclusive breastfeeding, children who were partially breastfed had a 4.2 times increased risk of death due to diarrheal disease. No breastfeeding was associated with a 14.2 times increased risk of death due to diarrheal disease in Brazilian children.

Infants in Bangladesh who were partially breastfed or not breastfed at all had a risk of acute respiratory infection death 2.4 times greater than exclusively breastfed infants. If children were predominantly breastfed, the risk of death due to acute respiratory infection was similar to that of exclusively breastfed children. The authors of this review discuss the impact of breastfeeding on child spacing, and estimate that exclusive breastfeeding can lead to decreased mortality of 20 percent when infants are spaced at least two years apart.

12. Increased Risk of Otitis Media and Ear Infections

The number of episodes of acute otitis media increased significantly with decreased duration and exclusivity of breastfeeding. U.S. infants who were exclusively breastfed for four months or more had a 50 percent reduction in episodes, compared to infants who were not breastfed. A 40 percent reduction of episodes was reported for breastfeeding infants who were supplemented before four months of age. Between six and twelve months of age, the incidence of first episodes of otitis media increased from 25 percent to 51 percent in infants exclusively breastfed. In infants that were exclusively formula-fed, the incidence rose from 54 percent to 76 percent during the second half of the first year. The authors concluded that breastfeeding, even for a short period (three months), would significantly reduce the episodes of otitis media during infancy.

13. Increased Risk of Side Effects of Environmental Contaminants

A Dutch study showed that at six years of age, cognitive development is affected by prenatal exposure to PCBs and dioxins. An adverse effect of prenatal exposure on neurological outcome was also demonstrated in the formula-fed group, but not in the breastfed group. Despite higher PCB exposures from breast milk, the study found at eighteen months, forty-two months, and six years of age that breastfeeding had a beneficial effect on the quality of movements, in terms of fluency, and in cognitive development tests.

The data gives evidence that prenatal exposure to PCBs has subtle negative effects on neurological and cognitive development of the child up to school age. The study also gives evidence that breastfeeding counteracts the adverse developmental effects of PCBs and dioxins.

How to Overcome Breastfeeding Barriers Checklist

❖ Be determined and steadfast in your resolve to breastfeed your baby. This can carry you a long way.

❖ Identify the barrier (e.g., fear, embarrassment, needing to return to work, etc.).

❖ Brainstorm ways to confront and overcome those barriers.

❖ Seek help.

❖ Make this your mantra: I think I can! I think I can!

❖ Remind yourself that only you can breastfeed your baby.

❖ Seek more help.

Chapter Five

It Takes Three

Including Dad in

the Breastfeeding Experience

You might ask yourself, "Why a chapter on fathers?" Well, it's simple. African American women are more likely to breastfeed and for a longer period of time if their mate is supportive; however, if he is not supportive, she will generally not last longer than a few days. This chapter will help you learn how to communicate with your mate about breastfeeding, share information about breastfeeding, as well as to educate a man about how to be an active and vital participant in the breastfeeding experience.

Rule #1: Include your Spouse/Boyfriend in Your Decision to Breastfeed.

Let's be honest here. When you're pregnant, it's all about you. Everyone wants to know how you're feeling, when are you due, will you have a boy or a girl, what you are craving, what they can do for you. Dad might get asked, "Do you want a son or a daughter?" That's just about it for him during nine months of pregnancy. Early on, you might ask him if he'd like to go with you when you have the sonogram, or perhaps if he wants the baby named after him. Or you'll fill him in on how much weight you're gaining, how tired and sick you are, how excited you are, where to pick up the ice cream and Chinese food you must have at one o'clock in the morning, or what colors you want him to paint the nursery. Again, Dad's feelings are often left out. Even when Dad is going to prenatal appointments and Lamaze sessions, he's rarely asked about what he wants or how he's feeling.

It's not that we deliberately leave him out. We just assume that because he's a man, he won't be interested in picking out nursery colors, or combing through lists of baby names, or seeing how the sonogram looks just like Grandma Jones. Society has led us to believe that men have more important, manly things to do. This could not be further from the truth.

Men tend to be more fact-oriented, while women are often more emotional. Men think with the left side of the brain, while women tend to think with the right side. Neither is better than the other, because both work together to make life balanced. So, when it comes to the decision on how to feed your baby, Dad should be a part of that process.

Step 1: Begin a Dialogue

As soon as you begin to receive information about infant-feeding options, you should set aside time to talk to the father about breastfeeding. Try to set a time when things are going well between you, and when he's particularly relaxed. It's easier to communicate when he's not busy or had a long day of work. Say, "We need to talk about how we're going to feed our baby." Then schedule some uninterrupted time to talk about breastfeeding. Start by telling him how important it is for the both of you to make this decision together. Use words like, "we," "us," "our baby," etc. to make him feel completely included in this decision. Be genuine when using words that make you include him in the family unity. You don't want to sound phony or pacifying.

You may even need to start telling yourself, "This baby is ours, not just mine. We are a family, which includes Dad, baby, and me." As nurturers, we naturally tend to take possession of the baby, wanting to protect him, but often protecting him from the very person he needs access to—Dad! If you are having these feelings, do a little self-talking. It will make a world of difference in your communication with your mate if you iron out your feelings of "it's just you and me, baby," to include your first "baby," who is your mate. Remember: you and your mate came first, before the baby. It will help you in the long run of your relationship if you let your mate know that you and he are on one team when it comes to parenting.

MAN TO MAN
From the Heart of Michael Covin

Before my wife became pregnant (which was in the first thirty days of marriage), I did not know anything about breastfeeding. I was of the members of society that would stare and think, *What is she doing?* So I now understand that I just lacked information and knowledge of the importance of breastfeeding. I was very involved in the prenatal period. I went to her appointments and we discussed what her needs were, as it pertains to a doctor vs. nurse midwife, and decided that the attention she required was going to come from a nurse midwife. We both participated in the birthing classes. I was not breastfed and believe that my mother felt formula-feeding was sufficient. This was before my children. Of course now she is a firm believer in the differences in a breastfed child.

What made me decide to support breastfeeding was information—something that African Americans do not seek nearly enough of. I have a saying, "What are you basing that on?" And if the person can provide me with actual information, I am willing to listen. My first daughter, Christian, was breastfed until two, and my youngest daughter, Logan,

(continued)

is currently being nursed at eight months old. My thoughts on extending breastfeeding are as follows. The child will stop when he or she is ready, and I am all about doing what is best for the child. People stop children from breastfeeding for their convenience. Many African American men do not support breastfeeding because of the lack of information, and because our society has men thinking the breast was created to attract them. The way to effectively reach men is to provide information. Maybe through articles from dads submitted to popular magazines (e.g., the page in *Essence* written by men). Maybe doing research on which popular Black families breastfed their children, and asking them to do public service announcements. Having a push for the African American Breastfeeding Alliance to grow and add more chapters, and to have a rotating meeting location. This will allow for different communities to be used as a forum for this information, thus increasing the chances of reaching more men. Also, the advocates of breastfeeding have to stop thinking that women are the only target for breastfeeding information, because if you can win the men you will get the women. Finally, I am an outspoken person. There is not a week that goes by that I don't mention breastfeeding to someone. I keep a breastfeeding pamphlet on my desk at work. I address the subject with pregnant women. When I see women with children, I ask them if they nursed the children. When I see formula, I speak out against it. I know that we are not challenging our community to step up and provide the best for our children, and in the end the community suffers. I am a firm believer that we have to move from doing what is convenient sometimes to doing what is best for the children. Thanks for allowing me to voice my opinion on such an important subject.

Step 2: Make Him Feel Important

Once you two sit down to discuss feeding options, ask, "What do you think about breastfeeding?" Don't say, "Do you think I should breastfeed?" or "Should I breastfeed or formula-feed?" These are called "closed-ended" questions, and won't get you very far into a conversation. They are closed-ended because they allow for a yes or no answer. If you ask, "Do you think I should breastfeed?" and he says, "No," there ends an open line of communication. If you ask, "Should I breastfeed or formula-feed?" he may pick one—yes or no—and that's the end of that. The point here is to start a dialogue with questions that will open the discussion up. For instance, starting with *how do you feel about,* or *what do you think about,* or *what are your thoughts on breastfeeding* works best. It will not allow for a one or two word answer. Even better than fostering a good start at communication, it shows your mate that you are interested in how he feels, and that his opinion is important in, and is a part of, this decision.

Then, once the dialogue has started, be a good listener. Don't keep your "eye on the prize," meaning, don't be so concerned that he supports breastfeeding that you don't give him time to talk. Let him finish sentences and statements without your input. Keep good eye contact with him so that he knows you are listening. A major problem in communication between men and women is that we don't stop to really listen to each other. We are so busy with our own agendas, needs, and desires that the other person becomes almost invisible.

If the conversation comes to a pause or lull, then you have the opportunity to support his feelings. This means that you let him know you affirm his feelings. Okay, maybe you're thinking, "He doesn't support breastfeeding, so no, I don't support his feelings." Well, the key here is not that you necessarily agree with him, but that you support his right to feel what he feels. Use statements like, "Yes, I understand why you'd feel that way," or "I feel you on that." It's not important that what he's saying makes no sense or is full of wrong information about breastfeeding. You're just trying to foster open communication.

At this point, the conversation (or part 2, 3, or 4 of the conversation at later dates) should be rolling along where you are listening to his feelings and the flow is comfortable. If at this point he has expressed a desire to support breastfeeding, move to step 4, otherwise, follow along with 3.

MAN TO MAN
Noel Barber, loving father to two children, and husband to me, the author

Prior to Kathi becoming pregnant, my knowledge of breastfeeding was very general. I knew that it was the best source of nutrition for a baby. I was not really aware of the specific benefits, the history, or the medical statistics that support the notion that breast milk is best. I was very involved in the prenatal period. I was exposed to breastfeeding in more detail during this time, and decided that it was the only option for our children, although I wasn't breastfed as a baby. First and foremost, I knew that it is the best source of nutrition for our child. Secondly, I felt like my support was a crucial part of my wife's successful breastfeeding experience. As with other life experiences, it was important for me to support and encourage her during the process. And it also saved us a lot of money!

Our children: Amyhr (now eight) was breastfed until the age of two, and Jayde (now six) was breastfed for seventeen months. I feel that each child should be dealt with individually. In our experience, my son had to be encouraged to stop breastfeeding, but my daughter decided to stop on her own. We made a collective decision to begin weaning my son around the age of two. It was a sensitive topic at the time. I realized that the (breastfeeding) bond between a woman and a child was intense for both of them. My wife was just as emotionally attached to the experience as my son was. It was a process of weaning the both of them. I think that breastfeeding adds to the amazing connection between a mother and child. I think that the health benefits for the baby, as well as the mother, should be provided for fathers in greater detail. Another major selling point should be the economic benefits. Providing this information should be a standard part of the prenatal process. It should be presented in writing as well as some other type of media (CD/video). It must be presented in a way that can capture the attention of Black men of all different backgrounds, family structures, and economic levels. Breastfeeding certainly added some "flavor" to the sexual experience that took some time getting used to. I can recall wondering if breastfeeding would reduce the sexual sensitivity of my wife's breasts after breastfeeding for about three consecutive years. I don't think it took us long to get used to being glazed over with breast milk after a sexual encounter. I have become a true advocate of breastfeeding since going through the process with my wife and children. I encourage women (especially minority women) to consider it, and have at times been asked to speak with expecting dads about the experience. To me, breastfeeding is simply a natural progression from childbirth. Witnessing the birth of my children and watching them being nourished naturally by my wife was a truly amazing experience. The benefits are so evident in the child. Some of my major observations of the benefits of breastfeeding are as follows:

(continued)

❖ Our children seldom had colds during the time they were breastfed.

❖ They never developed ear infections, which is common among infants.

❖ As our kids developed physically, they were always leaner than their peers.

I salute my wife for being so dedicated to our children, and our family.

Step 3: Go Deeper

Now you want to dig a little deeper into his feelings about breastfeeding. Keep in mind that most opinions about breastfeeding either come from a lack of good information, beliefs in myths, and/or a bad breastfeeding experience. Further, people who had any of the above may not initially realize that their lack of support of breastfeeding has deeper roots. Make statements like, "So you don't want me to breastfeed because you don't want me breastfeeding in public," or "You heard breastfeeding will make my breasts sag," or "Your mom didn't breastfeed you, and she said you did just fine on formula." By making these statements, you can make clear what he's saying. If you show that you understand what he's saying, then he'll say "yes" or "uh huh." If you've misunderstood and read the situation wrong, then he'll say, "No, that's not what I meant," or "What are you talking about?" This is good because it will keep the dialogue going and will clear up any problems in communicating his feelings. If you've got a good finger on his feelings about breastfeeding, then move on to step 4. If you're still not clear, then go back to asking open-ended questions and affirming his feelings to get to the root of what he's saying. This may take several discussions, so don't expect it all to happen at one time. If it does, bravo!

Step 4: Share the Knowledge

Once you understand his concerns, then you can begin sharing your breast-feeding knowledge. This will perhaps be the most exciting part of your exchange. Now you can share all the great information you've learned about breastfeeding.

Caution: Don't go on information overload. Don't pull out all your pamphlets, brochures, booklets, flyers, books, and videos. That will be overwhelming, and possibly put him on the defensive. You have to give him information in a way that he can receive it. If he's into reading, pass along a few highlighted chapters in this book, or give him a brochure or two. If he's more visual, and learns better by watching, share a video with him. However, during the first few discussions about breastfeeding, just share some major points about breastfeeding that will grab his attention and dispel myths. The following are some bite-size pieces of education to share with Dad that have been found to be particularly appealing to men:

❖ **Breast milk is free!** That's right. We can actually feed our baby for the first six months without it costing you one penny. You never have to add the "breastfeeding" item into your budget. In fact, breastfeeding can actually save us money. The more specialized the formula is, let's say soy-based or iron-fortified, the more expensive it will be. The average formula-feeding family can spend up to $400 or more a month on infant formula alone, not to mention even more money spent on bottles, bottle liners, nipples, etc. By breastfeeding, our family can actually save as much as $1,000 a year. This money can go toward savings for college, vacations, bills, and tickets to a basketball game—whatever you desire. Breastfeeding is not just an investment in our baby's health, but in our family's financial future.

❖ **Breast milk is best!** Why buy a hooptie if we can buy a Navigator or Benz? My milk can give our baby exactly what he'll need to have a near perfect start at life, as well as give him what he needs to grow for the first six months he's with us. It's the perfect food for his brain, so he can be whatever he wants to be later in life. Scientists did a study that found adults who had been breastfed as babies had higher IQs than adults who were formula-fed. Breast milk will protect him from germs and diseases, ear infections, obesity, diabetes, and other illnesses. We won't have to run back and forth to the doctor because breast milk will help him stay healthier. Black babies tend to die more, get sick more often, and have health problems like asthma, diabetes, and obesity that they have to deal with for a lifetime. We need to give him all we can, because as an African American child, he's going to need a head start.

❖ **Formula is not the same as breast milk.** I used to think that formula must be good since everyone uses it and it's supposed to be full of vitamins and minerals. But it's only been around for about one hundred years, and for the thousands of years before that, babies were fed breast milk. Formula is something scientists manufacture in a lab. And our baby is not a lab animal.

❖ **Formula companies don't really care about us.** Their main concern is to market their product. Formula companies make about two billion dollars a year. They spend money on advertisements and other things to make parents think infant formula is as good as breast milk, but it's not. It does not have anything in it that breast milk has. The ingredients in formula are copies or genetically engineered things that mimic breast milk. Formula companies also spend a lot of time marketing to African American communities to get us to use their products. They've done such a good job at selling us a bill of goods that we have the lowest breastfeeding rates and our babies are sicker than most other races. They send us free samples, coupons, and cool diaper bags to make it seem like they care about us. What they don't tell all the Black people they market to is that formula won't protect our babies from *anything*.

❖ **Breast milk will** *not* **make my breasts sag.** I don't know who came up with that, but the shape of my breasts will change during pregnancy because I'm getting larger. After the baby, my breasts will probably get even bigger because of the breast milk. They may change once I stop breastfeeding, but they would change even if I didn't breastfeed. Don't women who formula-feed their babies have sagging breasts after a few kids? So, my breasts have already started to change, and will probably change more as I grow older. But hopefully you'll love me no matter what, sagging or perky breasts. I'll still love you if you end up with a big belly and love handles.

❖ **Breastfeeding in public is** *not* **something to be embarrassed about.** I saw a mother nursing a baby in a crowd of people, and not only could you not see the woman's breast, but people kept going about their business—never even realizing the woman was breastfeeding. I can be discreet with it, and if worse comes to worst, I can breastfeed in the car, or in a store dressing room. I will not, though, breastfeed in a bathroom. It's dirty and germy. We don't each lunch or dinner there, so why should our baby? I think breastfeeding in public, discreetly, shows that I am a confident mom who is doing her "baby" thing!

Rule #2: Include Dad in the Breastfeeding Relationship.

You've agreed that you're going to breastfeed. Dad may still be concerned that he's going to be left out. He does not have to—and should not be— left out of the breastfeeding relationship. If it were not for him, there wouldn't be a baby to breastfeed in the first place! No, he won't be able to breastfeed the baby. That we simply can't accommodate. Yet, there are many other things he can do to be a part of this exciting time:

❖ **He can enjoy the love that breastfeeding creates.** There are few situations that come close to the miracle of childbirth. Breastfeeding, however, is pretty close. It's a miracle in itself to watch a baby latched on to his mother's breast, being nourished and nurtured at the same time. Breastfeeding creates hormones that stimulate feelings of love between you and your baby. This love is not lost on any bystander. Dad can sit with you and enjoy this wonderful time. He will be able to appreciate that, because of his support, your baby is getting something so special that will make him healthy and smart. Dad can look at you in a new light as the woman who is giving so much of herself for his baby. He may watch you overcome breastfeeding challenges and think, "She is truly amazing."

❖ **He can read all he can about breastfeeding.** This will not only reinforce the importance of breastfeeding, but will make him like your own in-house lactation consultant. Men are known for their ability to put things together and understand how things work. He could become extremely helpful in aiding you with problems.

❖ **He can help make you comfortable while breastfeeding**. By placing a pillow behind your back or under your feet.

❖ **If you pump your milk, he can organize the freezer to make sure your milk is labeled and stored safely.** He can also help with putting together your pump and keeping its parts clean. He can make sure that you are pumping regularly and that you have a good supply on hand. Bonus for him: being able to take the baby out with him for a few hours with a bottle of pumped breast milk, or being able to leave bottles for a baby-sitter so the two of you can go out for some much needed alone time.

- ❖ **Diapers. Diapers. Diapers.** Enough said.
- ❖ **Chores can become a shared activity, even if only for a short period of time.** Dad can help with laundry, cleaning around the house, folding clothes, vacuuming, washing dishes, cooking—the list is endless as you probably already know.
- ❖ **He can be a hands-on Dad.** He can pitch in and care for the baby when you need help, as long as he has a bottle of pumped breast milk. He can take the baby off your hands for a while for two purposes. One, so that you can get some much needed rest or to get your nails done, go to the mall, have coffee with friends, read a novel—whatever it is you like to do for you. Two, so that he and the baby can form a bond of their own, without your presence. While we are the primary nurturers, a father's role is indispensable. It's vital for your baby's future success that he/she be allowed to have a relationship with dad. Studies have shown that the presence of positive fathers can reduce the risk of suicide, high school drop-out rates, drug use, and other negative practices. A healthy relationship with a father, especially from birth, can give your child a good foundation to build on.
- ❖ **He can be a resource.** If you're too tense or stressed out about a breastfeeding situation, he can call and speak with the lactation consultant or doctor and get the help all of you need.

A final point to remember when including him in the breastfeeding relationship is to respond to his concerns about breastfeeding. You might think, "What does he have to be concerned about?" Well, since he is now a breastfeeding supporter, it's important to continue to listen to his concerns. In the beginning, he may be more focused on the needs of the baby. Is Junior getting enough milk or gaining enough weight? Is breast milk really all he needs? Shouldn't we be giving him water? Why is he still fussing after a feeding? All of these are normal concerns. Again, with some good listening skills, open dialogue, and education, you can put to rest many of these concerns.

After you, the baby, and Dad make it through the first few weeks of breastfeeding, overcoming challenges and getting into a groove, Dad's concerns will change. They'll tend to become more focused on his needs. He may feel a little left out, even after you've done everything on the list to include him. Just continue to reassure him that he is a part of it all. Most important, reassure him that he is a top priority for you.

When we have kids, we tend to place more emphasis on the children than on the relationship that created the children. It happens easily and quickly, and women cope with that change better and can hang with it for a long time. Fathers, however, come back to pre-kid memories quicker than we do. So, around the sixth week, right when you're about to have your six-week checkup that gives you the all-clear to return to sexual activity, Dad may begin to voice some of his own personal concerns about breastfeeding. He may not say, "Babe, I feel like the baby is getting more of your time than I am," or "I want some time with just you." You may have to read some nonverbal clues—and you know what to look for in his nonverbals. You can sense the change in his actions. It may not be for a few months that his concerns change. It may be around four to six months when he's had pressure from his mom that "The baby needs something else by now than just breast milk." It may be as the baby approaches his first birthday that weaning is a major concern for him. Interestingly, men tend to be more verbal in their communication about the time the baby "is supposed to" stop breastfeeding. It becomes easier for him to say, "I think the baby needs to stop breastfeeding," than for him to say, "I want more of you."

Again, all of these concerns are valid, even if they seem way out in left field to you. We feel what we feel, regardless of any truths involved. Communication and affirmation of his feelings are key if you are going to continue having his support of breastfeeding. There is no quick fix here. The main thing for you to do is stay calm, address his concerns, and love him anyway.

Finally, let's talk about sex. Dad is a true breastfeeding supporter. He's even asking his pregnant coworker in the cubicle next to his, "Hey, are you going to breastfeed your baby? When Junior comes, he's going to be a champ because of breast milk." You have the baby. Once you feel comfortable enough to, and your body is healed, you and your man know that "tonight is the night." The baby has had a bath, been fed, and is sleeping soundly in the crib—for a good two-hour stretch. Clothes are off and the hormones that created baby number one have kicked in. And squirt, there is a steady stream of breast milk spraying dad with a purpose. You stop, look at the milk, then at each other and fall off the bed laughing hysterically. Neither of you have ever seen anything like it. You're thinking, "Okay, I guess this night is done." He's thinking, "Let's get back to it." Oddly, the same hormone that creates your letdown is the same one that stimulates orgasms. Oxytocin kicks off two totally different responses for some of life's greatest experiences, breastfeeding and orgasm. Be prepared for him to potentially have a little issue with leaking breasts during sex, or his own swallows of breast milk. Or, he may not even blink. If he doesn't have a problem, and you don't either, just go with the flow. If he does take issue with leaking breasts, then try to talk about it openly. Usually, breast leakage stops after a few weeks or months. It's different for each woman. Generally, the leaking simply takes a little getting used to, but after a few funny moments, you both can continue to enjoy your sex life. If Dad refuses sex because of leaking breasts, perhaps you should consider talking with a therapist, because chances are the breast milk is not the true issue.

Top Four Concerns Dad May Have and How to Address Them

1. Concern: Breastfeeding makes your breasts sag.

Response: The shape of breasts starts to change as early as age nine and will continue to change through puberty, pregnancy, breastfeeding, menopause, and old age. It's not the breastfeeding that does it. Gaining and losing weight will make a difference in the shape of breasts, too. Women who never breastfeed their children and women who never have children at all get sagging breasts, too.

2. Concern: I don't want you to breastfeed in public with people looking at your breasts.

Response: Lots of women breastfeed in public and no one ever knows it. That's because it can be done discreetly by using a receiving blanket or other covering where the breasts can't be seen at all. (Demonstrate with a doll to show him how it can be done.)

3. Concern: Formula is good for the baby because it's full of vitamins and minerals.

Response: Formula does not provide any protection against disease, illness, and germs that the baby is exposed to. Formula is also full of fat that can lead to an overweight baby. Breast milk provides everything the baby will need to grow and be healthy long into childhood. It also protects the baby from ear infections, colds, diarrhea, lung infections, allergies, diabetes, childhood cancer, sudden infant death syndrome (SIDS), bacteria, viral infections, and many other illnesses. Breast milk also boosts the baby's brain.

4. Concern: I'll be left out if you breastfeed the baby.

Response: No way! Your support will make it a good experience for all of us. You can help the baby learn how to drink my breast milk from a bottle when I have to go out or go back to work. You can take the baby out, between feedings, so I can get some things done, or to have a break. You can help with diapers and playing with the baby. You can help chores get done faster. Most important, you can be a proud father that our baby is getting a special treasure with benefits that will last a lifetime.

COMMUNICATION TIPS

By keeping the following ideas in mind, you can have a good chance at positive communication between you and your mate. Remember that good communication may not happen overnight, but can be greatly improved over time with effort by both of you. Communication takes two.

- ❖ **Be respectful.** Communication will fail if your mate feels you don't respect him or are trying to control him.
- ❖ **Change your language.** From "you" statements to "we" or "our."
- ❖ **Give your undivided attention.** There's nothing worse than trying to communicate feelings when the other person is preoccupied. Don't have the breastfeeding discussion(s) while doing two or three other things. Talking while doing laundry or cooking dinner should be fine though.
- ❖ **Praise him!** Recent studies have shown that men need affirmation. They may not ask for it, like we do, but they need it nonetheless. Imagine how open you feel to discuss certain things when you've been given compliments or praises from your man. The same

(continued)

will work for him. Thank him for how hard he works for the family, or how he keeps the lawn up, or how great he will be as a father. Whether big or small, praises boost the male ego and can open many doors for you, and not just communication!

❖ **Be direct and don't assume.** Has your mate ever said, "I didn't know that was what you wanted. I can't read your mind." As women, we tend to be more intuitive and can connect the dots to understand underlying feelings and emotions. Well, men are more direct and they don't even try to read our minds. They appreciate it when we are direct so that there is no guesswork about what we like, want, or feel. Notice how relaxed and easy-going male to male relationships are—they tend to have long-term friendships without a lot of ups and downs because they are straightforward and don't get involved in guessing games. Tell him exactly how you feel and you'll gain his respect.

Facts about Breastfeeding for Dads
Why You Should Support Breastfeeding

What's in It for You?
❖ You can be the proud father of a healthy, smart, happy, African American baby.
❖ You can save your family hundreds of dollars a year—money that can be used for college savings, vacations, bills, whatever you want!
❖ You can get more rest because you won't have to get up in the middle of the night to make bottles.
❖ You can experience the special love and bonding that breastfeeding creates.

What's in It for Your Baby?

❖ A head start in life. Not only will your baby be healthier than his peers from birth and long into childhood, but chances are he'll be smarter, too.

❖ All the vitamins, minerals, and nutrients needed for the first six months of life.

❖ Protection, each time he breastfeeds, from asthma, ear infections, diabetes, diarrhea, allergies, childhood cancer, and respiratory infections.

❖ A better chance to reach his first birthday because breastfeeding protects against sudden infant death syndrome (SIDS).

What's in It for Mom?

❖ Faster return to her prepregnancy weight. Go on, you can smile at that one!

❖ Better health: protection from ovarian cancer, which is on the rise in our community, and premenopausal breast cancer. African American women die more from breast cancer than white women.

❖ Less chance of excessive bleeding and infection after delivery.

❖ Increased self-confidence.

Sample Dialogue

Renee: *Have you ever thought about how we're going to feed the baby?*

James: *What do you mean?*

Renee: *I mean, are we going to feed the baby breast milk or formula?*

James: *Oh. I haven't really thought about it. Formula, I guess.*

Renee: *Why formula?*

James: *I don't know. That's what my sister gives her son. It's good for them, right?*

Renee: *Actually, I've been reading a lot about formula and it's not as good as they make it seem on commercials.*

James: *So…what? You're thinking about breastfeeding?*

Renee: *Sort of, but I wanted to talk about it with you. I want this to be something we decide together.*

James: *That's cool, but nobody breastfeeds anymore. My mother didn't even breastfeed me.*

Renee: *I know. My mother didn't breastfeed me either, but I have learned some things you wouldn't believe about breastfeeding.*

James: *Yeah, I know. You come home with some new information about pregnancy and babies almost every day. But breastfeeding? I just don't know.*

Renee: *Let's talk about it, then. How do you feel about breastfeeding?*

James: *Like I said, I never thought about it before. I don't even think I've ever seen anyone doing it. Plus, I heard it'll make your breasts sag.*

Renee: *I've never seen anyone breastfeeding before either. And I think the breast sagging thing is just a myth. I mean, look at my girl Faye. She has three kids, didn't breastfeed any of them, and her breasts are definitely heading south.*

James: *You got me on that one. So, why are you thinking about it?*

Renee: *I think we both want what's best for the baby, right?*

James: *That's right. Nothing's too good for my baby.*

Renee: *From what my doctor said and what I learned in my prenatal classes, breast milk is the best.*

James: *Hmmm.*

Renee then shares information she's learned about breastfeeding.

Dad's Breastfeeding Math

Dad + Mom = Love and Baby
Breast Milk + Baby = Healthy Baby
Breast Milk + Baby's Brain = High IQ
High IQ + African American Baby = Brighter Future
Breast Milk + Baby = More $$$

Man to Man

Ira James is a forty-two-year-old father of five children, ranging in age from thirteen years down to eleven months. He, his wife, Kim, of fifteen years, and their children reside in Los Angeles. Ira, a native Haitian who spent most of his life in New York, is currently in graduate school for his MBA. He enjoys creating culinary masterpieces with his catering business. He is also a respected mentor of young boys in his community.

Kathi: *What were your thoughts about breastfeeding before your wife became pregnant?*

Ira: *Breastfeeding is accepted in my West Indian culture, and long recognized as the healthiest way to nourish a baby.*

Kathi: *How involved were you during the prenatal periods of your wife's pregnancies?*

Ira: *I was very involved, and with each pregnancy. I would speak with the baby, massage Mom's stomach and lower back, and usually went to prenatal visits.*

Kathi: *Were you breastfed?*

(continued)

Ira: *Again, cultural mores supported it, so I was breastfed. My mother really shared many of these experiences.*

Kathi: *What made you decide to support breastfeeding?*

Ira: *Literature and La Leche League support groups encouraged us to breastfeed.*

Kathi: *How long were your children breastfed?*

Ira: *With five children, my wife has been breastfeeding off and on for more than thirteen years. Each child was breastfed for an average of three years.*

Kathi: *Wow! How do you feel about your children being breastfed past one or two years?*

Ira: *It's simple. It's natural, healthy, and fosters parental bonding.*

Kathi: *As you know, many Black men don't support breastfeeding. What do you think can be done to communicate the importance of breastfeeding?*

Ira: *We really need to communicate the truth, the risks of using infant formula, and we need more literature that manifests the overwhelming health benefits of breastfeeding.*

Chapter Six

Take the Stress Out of Going Back to Work
Plan Ahead

More than 75 percent of African American women have to return to work before their baby is two months old. The myth that you have to stop breast-feeding once you return to work is one of the biggest barriers facing African American women. It's one of the major reasons we stop breastfeeding so early. Is it worth the effort? How does it work? I don't have my own office. Where do I buy a breast pump? Where do I pump? I don't think my boss will like this. My friend said she wasn't able to pump enough milk to leave with the sitter.

These are all typical concerns that many women have when faced with breastfeeding and returning to work. There are a number of important reasons why you should continue to breastfeed, even after you return to work. First, it's recommended by the American Academy of Pediatrics and doctors, that all babies be fed only breast milk for the first six months of life to ensure optimal health. These benefits continue long into childhood, and even adult years. Breastfeeding should then be continued for the first year of life, along with solid foods, and longer for even more benefits.

If your maternity leave is between six and twelve weeks, like most women, then you can see why continuing to breastfeed is vital for your baby's health. When your baby enters a child care setting, he will be exposed to a number of potentially life-threatening germs. If you continue breastfeeding, your baby will likely be protected from most of these, or will have a less severe incident of an illness. If you stop breastfeeding, your baby will be left open, without any protection from illness that can be severe, even requiring hospitalization or worse, since infant formula does not provide protection of any sort.

Second, you won't have to worry about taking a lot of time off from work because your baby will be healthy. This does not mean that your baby will never get sick or that you'll never have to take off work to care for him, but your chances of having to deal with either instance will be lower than that of your coworkers who don't breastfeed their babies.

Third, breastfeeding can help you to continue to feel close to your baby once you go back to work. For many women, it is a stressful, often depressing thought to have to leave their infant with a sitter—be it a friend, family member, or stranger. After weeks of cuddling, holding, kissing, and bonding, it is a challenging, and often traumatic, task to leave the baby and return to work. The hormones of lactation, oxytocin and prolactin, can help you to continue that bond with your baby. These hormones actually produce feelings of love and longing for your baby. When you see your baby at the end of the workday or shift, you will reconnect in a way that only breastfeeding provides. Plus, these hormones will continue to work for you by helping you to relax and ease away the tension from work.

Fourth, the longer you breastfeed, the greater the health benefits are for you. You read earlier that breastfeeding reduces your chances of getting ovarian cancer, premenopausal breast cancer, and osteoporosis. This is particularly important for women in our community because breast cancer is one of the leading causes of death for African American women. The longer you breastfeed, the greater protection you have from this deadly disease. Breastfeeding also helps to reduce postpartum depression, which can hinder your life at home and at work. And you can continue to burn up to a thousand calories a day by continuing your breastfeeding.

Finally, breastfeeding can help to increase your self-esteem and leave you feeling empowered. This is especially important if you don't have a leadership or management position at work, or if your employer does not support its staff. You can feel confident at work because you're doing something for your child that will benefit him for a lifetime. This can keep you confident that you are making a difference in the world!

With good planning, you can successfully return to work without disturbing your breastfeeding experience. Please know in advance that pumping at work will take some time to get used to, but you can do it! If you can survive childbirth and the first eight weeks of breastfeeding, you can take on the world. There are some key areas to consider before you have the baby, including talking with your employer, learning about breast pumps and milk storage, and finding a breastfeeding-friendly child-care provider.

Your Employer

You may be thinking, "What in the world does my boss have to do with me breastfeeding?" The fact is, your employer can have a crucial role in your breastfeeding experience once you return to work. Let's look at why. There are two main things you'll need from your employer once you go back to work. You'll need the time to pump your breast milk, and a sanitary, private place to pump. Unfortunately, employers are not required by law in every state to give you the time or place to pump your milk. Communicating with your supervisor and/or Human Resources manager is important to make your pumping experience a success. Asthmatics are allowed time to get treatments during the day. Diabetics are given time for insulin regiments. These and other health-related practices are necessary. Coffee drinkers are permitted time to make fresh pots of coffee throughout the day, while talking around the coffee maker. Office parties and celebrations of all sorts are planned during the work day. Smokers slip out to stand right in front of the office to smoke throughout the day. Employers approve of, support, and often look the other way in the face of these practices.

This is not meant as a soapbox against any of the above practices. These are normal routines that occur in offices and workplaces across the country. Yet, while employers look the other way as smokers head out several times a day, women who seek time to pump milk are often frowned upon in the workplace. Why shouldn't a woman trying to provide the best for her baby be supported in the same regard as a person with a health issue, an office planner, smoker, or coffee drinker?

Since so few women are breastfeeding once they return to work—especially women in our community—there is little precedence for breast-feeding women in the workplace. This is why it's critical for you to have a discussion with your employer before you go on maternity leave. If you start early on in your pregnancy, then you give yourself a good window of time to convince your employer that you should be supported. Think about it. You already know that breast milk is the best form of nutrition for babies, and that babies should be breastfed for at least six months. Since most women have an average of six weeks of maternity leave, how can your baby still get what he'll need when you return to work?

Your employer may not, initially, be a breastfeeding supporter. Perhaps she: hasn't had a baby, didn't breastfeed, had a bad breastfeeding experience, or has no information on the importance of breastfeeding. Perhaps he: is older and breastfeeding was only for "lower-class women" in his day, watched his wife suffer from severe pain while breastfeeding, or thinks that a baby-related issue shouldn't be handled in the office. You may be up against these and many other opinions and experiences about breastfeeding.

Don't assume that since you know how important breastfeeding is, your employer will as well.

Before the Talk

Do your homework. Your boss will to want know what's in it for the company. See, breastfeeding your baby does not rank high on the list of priorities for your place of business. Time is money for all companies. Even time off for maternity leave is seen as damaging to a company's productivity. Let's face it: we don't live in the most mother/baby/family–friendly country. A simple look at our maternity leave practices proves that fact. In many European countries, women are given extended, paid maternity leave to care for their babies. We get a measly six weeks to be with a newborn, or twelve if we have the time saved up or use the Family Leave Act. So, it will be important for you to be prepared to share with your boss how supporting a breastfeeding staff member can positively affect the workplace. Here are points that you can share with your employer about the benefits of having a breastfeeding member on the team.

❖ **Less absenteeism.** Breastfed babies are healthier than their formula-fed peers. Women who breastfeed tend to take off less time from work to take care of sick babies because of the health benefits of breast milk. This means fewer calls at the start of a shift to say "I can't come in because my baby is sick." Even men whose wives are breastfeeding will have to take off less time to care for a sick child. When a staff person has to take a day (or more) off, it affects other workers' productivity as well. She'll tend to be distracted throughout her day, again affecting company productivity. Think about this…an employee will take an average of: one to two days off for a child with an ear infection; two to three days off for a child with complications from the ear infection; one to two days off for a child with allergies;

and two to seven, or more, days for a child with pneumonia, asthma, bronchiolitis, or other respiratory infections.

❖ **Increased morale.** There are few things more productive than a happy worker. When employees know that their employer cares about them and their family, they are apt to be punctual, more devoted to the company, and willing to go the extra mile. When staffers benefit from the company's provision for a personal matter, they will share that information with their coworkers. A happy work environment is contagious, and can mean increased productivity across the board. By supporting a breastfeeding employee, the company shows its concern for family.

❖ **Healthier workforce.** When people have to take off work to care for an ill child, they are left open to potentially contagious disease. So, if their child has a contagious illness, they will likely contract it. This will increase the likelihood of a day or more off from work. Even worse, they may come to work sick, spreading germs to their coworkers. This can lead to additional absenteeism from other employees, and a potential outbreak of the flu, stomach virus, or other illness.

❖ **Positive reputation.** It can benefit a company in many ways to be seen as family-friendly. Quality people have strong family values. They will want to work there because the management cares, not just about their employees, but their families too. Breastfeeding equals family. A family-friendly image can spark media attention, which can increase revenue, because so few companies can proudly say they are. This image makes a strong statement that families matter.

Introducing Your Baby to the Bottle

You can safely begin to introduce your baby to bottle use after breastfeeding and your breast milk has been established, when you and baby are nursing well, and the baby is growing. A general rule of thumb is that bottles should not be introduced before the baby is four to six weeks old. Some babies will use a bottle and breastfeed interchangeably from birth, for many reasons: health, early return to work, or cultural practices. However, to alleviate any potential problems, such as nipple confusion or disrupting your milk supply, it's best to wait at least four weeks to get breastfeeding off to a good start.

What is the best type of bottle to use? Well, there are a number of artificial nipples on the market that claim to be "just like mother's nipple." You can't duplicate nature! So you'll have to test nipples by trial and error. Some babies will like more expensive, latex nipples, while others will be comfortable using ones found at the dollar store. As long as the nipple is sterile, your baby will let you know which one works best for him.

Try introducing a bottle of breast milk when he is content. Don't attempt this if he is screaming hungry or not feeling well. You want him to be open to something new. Be aware that it's likely he won't take the bottle from you initially. Dad, Grandma, another family member, or friend can help you here. You may even have to leave the room. Your baby's senses are strongly attached to you. If he even smells you in the room, he may refuse the bottle altogether. It will take several attempts to get him used to using a bottle because drinking from it is different than at the breast. Perhaps run an errand after he seems to warm up to the idea of using a bottle. When you get back, and he's taken up to two ounces of milk, you can begin to feel confident that he'll be able to take more breast milk from the bottle. Rest assured, he won't starve himself!

There are some babies who are strong willed and refuse to use any type of artificial nipple. This is another reason why you should try introducing the bottle a few weeks before you return to work. Some babies will put up a good fight. Keep offering the bottle, but also introduce an alternative to bottle-feeding, such as a spoon or cup. This can be more time consuming and messy, but not impossible. You may want to contact a breastfeeding peer counselor, lactation consultant, or nurse to help you learn how to feed this way effectively.

Choosing a Breast Pump

You've decided to keep breastfeeding after you return to work. Now, what type of breast pump will you need? That depends on a number of factors, including how long you will be away from your baby during the day/night, and your finances. Breast pumps range in price from under $30 to well over $200. The lower priced ones are for minimal pumping while the more expensive ones are for maximum pumping potential. Many hospitals and companies offer low-cost breast pump rentals. When making your decision about rental or purchase, consider how many children you plan to have. Depending on your financial situation, if you plan to have and breastfeed more than one child, it may be a good investment to purchase a quality electric breast pump.

Types of Breast Pumps

Hand or Manual

Hand or manual expressing of breast milk is useful when you have limited pumping needs, say for an occasional separation, or for one missed feeding a day. It's useful to help soften your areola if you're engorged. It's also helpful to have a manual pump, or learn to use your own hands to express milk if you've forgotten your breast pump, it won't work, there is not outlet available, or you can't purchase one yet. Manual breast pumps generally cost under $30.

Electric Breast Pumps

These pumps are designed for women who will be away from their babies for longer periods of time. They work by either pumping one or both breasts at the same time. Their suction emulates, but does not replace, the way your baby suckles at your breast. These pumps range in price from $50 (which I don't recommend because they could be of low quality and potentially damaging) to $250. Breast pump companies include Bailey, Medela, and Ameda. Pumps can be purchased at your local baby store, or even in your hospital.

Sample Letter to Employer

This letter should be given to your employer with modifications as you see fit to meet the needs of your work environment. A copy of this book would be a nice addition as well. You can say it's a gift to the entire staff as a resource book to remain the property of the company. You can also download literature from the Internet about the importance of breastfeeding, and how companies benefit from supporting their breastfeeding staff. Set up a meeting if you can, with your employer, or send this via interoffice mail. Be open about what you want and use this letter and book as back-up.

Dear Employer,

We know that you are concerned about the well-being of your employees and their role in increased productivity, morale, and business services. That is why we are writing to invite your participation in an important worksite endeavor, the development of worksite support for breastfeeding employees. Many organizations have come together across the country to support breastfeeding: U.S. Department of Health and Human Services, American Academy of Pediatrics (AAP), Maternal and Child Health

Bureaus, Centers for Disease Control, African American Breastfeeding Alliance, La Leche League, and many, many other experts and medical professionals. These experts share the belief that breastfeeding is beneficial to individuals, families, employers, and the nation.

Why is breastfeeding important? Breast milk is the perfect food for a newborn's growth and brain development. It protects them from many illnesses, from ear infections to sudden infant death syndrome to respiratory viruses and obesity. Breastfeeding protects the mother from many forms of cancer, as well as helps her to lose weight faster, and increases her self-confidence. It saves the country millions of dollars a year in health care costs from caring for sick babies.

When an employee returns from maternity leave, she wants to be a productive and profitable employee, and a good mother. That is why so many women today are choosing to breastfeed their babies, even as they return to work. They understand that breastfeeding keeps babies healthy and helps them grow to their optimal potential. The protective health benefits of breastfeeding positively and directly affect the employer through worker productivity, improved employee morale, and decreased health care costs. National studies indicate that women who breastfeed are more productive on the job, worry less about their babies, and miss fewer work hours due to illness in themselves and their babies.

Many companies across the country support their breastfeeding employees by providing time, space, and even breast pumps for their breastfeeding employees. The following companies are recognized for their support of mothers with families. These include: Starbucks, Aetna Insurance Company, Kodak, Cigna, and First Chicago National Bank.

How can you support your breastfeeding employees? The process of continuing to breastfeed and returning to work can be made more efficient with your help in providing the small investment of the following:

❖ *Time for breaks to pump her milk, perhaps two fifteen- to twenty-minute sessions—the same amount of time smokers and coffee drinkers take freely, and without benefit to the company. Or allow her to split her lunch break into two sessions.*

❖ *A clean and private place for employees to pump breast milk during breaks. This could be an unused office, storage, or conference room. It just requires a space, near a restroom, with a comfortable chair and an outlet for the breast pump.*

❖ *Refrigeration—important and suggested, but not required. Pumped breast milk should be refrigerated. A mini-refrigerator would serve this purpose and keep breast milk in a safe, sterile, and separate location from other refrigeration needs.*

❖ *Breastfeeding resource materials. Breastfeeding information workshops by your HR department for expecting parents.*

❖ *Optional: Some employers even offer an on-the-job breast pump, or low cost pump rentals. Others offer extended maternity leave, up to six months. Many employers are exploring flex-time options, job sharing, telecommuting, part-time work hours, on-site child care, and other creative measures to continue job productivity while supporting breastfeeding and maternal care. Now that's going the extra mile for the employee.*

❖ *It's that simple!*

Thank you for being a leader in your community. If you would like more information, please feel free to contact the African American Breastfeeding Alliance at (877) 532-8535.

STORING BREAST MILK

Breast milk can be kept safe, fresh, and full of all its important nutrients and antibodies by following these important guidelines. You should know that it's normal for your pumped breast milk to look different after refrigeration or freezing. Don't be alarmed, this is absolutely normal. The color may change from white to a bluish or yellowish tinge. It will often separate, and you'll notice a creamy layer on top and milk at the bottom. Breast milk is so incredible that its antibodies can help it to stay fresh, even without refrigeration, but for maximum safety always refrigerate or freeze your breast milk. Fresh, or just pumped, breast milk can be kept:

❖ For six to twelve months in a deep freezer (0°F or less)

❖ For three to four months in a freezer attached to a refrigerator (0°F)

❖ Up to two weeks in a freezer inside a refrigerator

❖ Up to eight days in a refrigerator (32°F–39°F)

❖ Up to ten hours at room temperature (66°F–72°F)

❖ Once thawed, breast milk can be kept for one hour at room temperature and twenty-four hours in a refrigerator

Storage Containers

To ensure that your breast milk is kept safe, sterile, and free of freezer burn or other contamination, yet maintain its valuable ingredients, choose your milk storage containers carefully. The following containers are considered safe for your breast milk:

- ❖ Glass or plastic with tight fitting lids (sterilize by washing with warm, soapy water, and then allowing time to air dry).
- ❖ Breast milk storage bags (tend to be more durable and will hold up well in the freezer).
- ❖ Disposable bottle bags (tend to be less durable and may break open in the freezer, potentially causing freezer burn and or contamination).

Other important tips to consider for safely storing your breast milk

- ❖ To provide extra protection to this most precious commodity, a good practice is to double bag all of your breast milk in freezer or storage bags.
- ❖ To prevent waste, only put two to four ounces of milk in each container because your breast milk will expand in the freezer once frozen.

Thawing Breast Milk

Breast milk should never be thawed or heated in a microwave. It can burn your baby's mouth because there may be "hot areas" of milk in the bottle, as microwaving may not cause even heat throughout. Also, if you microwave breast milk, it can destroy the unique and precious antibodies your baby needs. To thaw breast milk, follow these guidelines:

- ❖ Place container of breast milk in a bowl of warm water for about thirty seconds, and shake periodically for even distribution of warmth.

(continued)

❖ You can also hold the container under warm running water.

❖ You can also heat—not boil—water for thawing in a pan, but don't place the container into the pot. This can make the milk too hot for your baby, and potentially cause burns.

❖ Thawed, not heated, breast milk can be kept in the refrigerator for up to twenty-four hours.

❖ To defrost, place frozen breast milk in the refrigerator for eight to twelve hours.

❖ Once heated, throw out any breast milk not used during a feeding.

Labeling Stored Breast Milk

You'll want to label your refrigerated and frozen breast milk. Labeling will help you to keep track of how long your milk has been refrigerated or frozen. You may think, "Oh, I'll know how long it's been there." It's not quite that simple. With the demands of a baby, other small children, boyfriend/husband, work, hobbies, friends, religious activities, it will be almost impossible to keep track of each bottle of milk. Just think about how many times you've looked in the freezer and can't remember how old some frozen meat is? You'll want to use the oldest stored breast milk first. For instance, if you nurse your baby past eight months, you'll need to know if the frozen milk is too old to use. Many of the breast milk storage bags have a space on them to write the date the milk was stored. Disposable bottle bags can easily be labeled with an ink pen or marker as well.

Tips for the Transition Back to Work

❖ **Do make your decision early.** Don't decide that you're going to keep breastfeeding two days before you return to work. You'll need at least two to four weeks to get your baby used to an artificial nipple, and you'll have to get into the practice of pumping your milk.

❖ **Do begin to pump your breast milk at least three weeks before going back to work.** This will give you a supply of breast milk to start from. Pump whenever possible—early in the morning, throughout the day, and even pump on one breast while nursing your baby on the other side. Pump on the weekends and on other days off, as well as during the night, and whenever your breasts feel full. This will increase your milk supply and help to maintain it once you return to work.

❖ **Do prioritize breastfeeding.** Make breastfeeding the last thing you do before you go to work and the first thing you do when you see your baby. This will again help with maintaining your milk supply.

❖ **Do plan ahead.** Cook more than one dinner on the weekends and freeze them so that you don't have to rush home to cook every night after work. Get clothes, including diaper bag, items for siblings, lunch, and even breakfast ready or prepared the night before. Or, like mothers of old used to do: wash, fold, and iron all laundry for the week during the weekend. These tips can save you anywhere from fifteen to sixty extra minutes each morning, time that can be used for extra sleep, meditation, pumping, or breastfeeding.

❖ **Do have a picture of the baby with you while you're pumping.** This will help to stimulate your letdown, "tricking" your body into thinking the baby is there.

❖ **Do try to relax while you are pumping during the day.** Stress can slow down or completely stop your milk from flowing. Look at pictures of your baby and think about him. Call your day care provider, if possible, before you pump, to hear the familiar sounds of your baby. Use creative visualization. Here's how. Close your eyes. Take deep breaths, inhaling and exhaling slowly through your nose. Imagine yourself breastfeeding your baby. Think about the great benefits you're giving him with your breast milk.

❖ **Don't skip breakfast, or any other meal.** Working mothers tend to forget their health in the process of caring for the family. Even a quick bowl of cereal or a few pieces of fruit will give you some extra energy and valuable nutrients your body will need. Eating a well-balanced diet is essential for your health, and to replenish your body from breastfeeding.

❖ **Don't start back to work on a Monday.** Many people find Mondays overwhelming—the beginning of the work week looms with seen and unseen events. That said, starting back to work at the end of the week, Thursday or Friday, will be less stressful. It will also allow you the chance to try out your new routine. You'll see what it's like to get things ready for the baby, dropping him off at day care, and pumping during the day.

❖ **Don't use bottles when you're at home with the baby.** Breastfeed your baby frequently to keep up your milk supply.

❖ **Do expect the unexpected.** No matter how detailed and organized your planning is, you cannot anticipate everything. Leave room in your mind for unexpected events that could potentially disrupt your day, like a last minute diaper change when you're running late, or a hole in your stockings, a lost bus pass, an empty gas tank. If you take these little things in stride, you can laugh and proceed confidently with your day.

> ## Breastfeeding-Friendly Companies
>
> | | |
> |---|---|
> | Kodak | National Semiconductor |
> | Starbucks Coffee | Eddie Bauer |
> | Cigna | PNC Financial Services Group |
> | Menasha | Crouse & Co. |
> | First Chicago National Bank | |

How to Pump Your Breast Milk

Always begin with clean hands and a clean breast pump.

❖ Sit in a comfortable position, using a pillow for your back, or a footstool—whatever works for you.

❖ Read the complete instructions of your breast pump's manufacturer. Watch the enclosed user video if one is available.

❖ Place the flange onto your breast, with your nipple in the center of the hole. If your nipple is touching any side of the flange, stop and start over. If not, once you begin pumping, the suction can damage your nipple and cause extreme pain. By having your nipple at the center of the flange, then you can get the optimal use of your breast pump.

❖ Set your pump, if using an electric one, at the lowest, most effective setting. By setting it too high, you can cause yourself undue pain and potential nipple damage. Conversely, by setting it too low, you may not get enough pressure to get your milk flowing.

❖ If you're using a manual pump, squeeze the handle or lever rapidly and pause, then repeat, much like your baby nursing at the breast. This will help to stimulate the letdown and get your milk flowing.

❖ At home, pump as often as possible. At work, pump two to three times a day, if possible.

Your Child-Care Provider's Role in Breastfeeding

Believe it or not, everyone may not understand the importance of breast-feeding, even those whose business it is to care for babies. It is a general assumption by many women that child-care providers won't be concerned with caring for a breastfed baby. Nothing could be further from the truth! The fact is there are child-care providers who are uncomfortable with handling breast milk. Why? Because it's a bodily fluid and some fear being exposed to it. Be aware that your child-care provider may not have breast-fed, and may not have dealt with a breastfed child before. Your baby will be used to a loving, nurturing lifestyle fostered through breastfeeding. It will be important for you to select a child-care provider who is breastfeeding-friendly, or at least open to learning more.

There is little difference in caring for a breastfed and formula-fed infant in the child care setting. The main distinction comes with handling and thawing breast milk. Also, the breastfed infant may need to be changed more often as breast milk is more easily digested than formula.

Child-care providers, albeit in a home or a center environment, work on a schedule for optimal child care service. This is important to manage the number of kids they have to care for; generally there is a two (in home) or four (center setting) infant-to-staff-member ratio. Thus, any deviation in the provider's routine could be a potential cause for concern.

Choosing a Child-Care Provider

You should begin your search for a child-care provider as soon as you find out you're pregnant. This will give you ample time to sift through the different types of providers available to you. The child-care industry is a busy one. Keep in mind that many providers, both in-home and center-based, have waiting lists; and often the infant spots go quickly.

It's okay for you to interview child-care providers. In fact, it's a necessity.

This person, or people, will be caring for your baby an average of eight hours per day. They will spend more time with your child than most of your family members! They will play a major role in your baby's development and growth. Here's a quick checklist on what to look for in a child-care provider:

- ❖ current, state-certified child care license
- ❖ clean, safe environment (no chipping paint on the walls or loose floorboards)
- ❖ clean toys and bathroom
- ❖ daily schedule of activities
- ❖ child care philosophy
- ❖ open policy for parents to "drop-in"

Here is a list of questions for you to ask potential child-care providers. Feel free to add and delete from this list as needed. Ask your friends about their experience in locating good child care. They can offer advice on child-care providers to avoid, as well.

- ❖ How do you feel about breastfeeding?
- ❖ If you don't support it, are you willing to learn more about breast-feeding?
- ❖ Are you willing to follow the simple steps to thaw and warm breast milk?
- ❖ Will you allow me to pop in during my lunch break, or other times if possible, to breastfeed the baby?
- ❖ Will you hold off on feeding the baby close to the time I am to pick him up?
- ❖ Will you provide loving care for this child?
- ❖ What is your emergency and fire policy?
- ❖ Can I see your list of daily activities?
- ❖ Tell me about the other children and families in the center.

Important Tips for Your Child-Care Provider

❖ Wash hands before handling stored breast milk.

❖ Thaw milk in a bowl of warm water or under warm running water.

❖ Do not microwave or boil breast milk.

❖ Keep stored breast milk labeled with the baby's name and date, in a safe part of the refrigerator so it won't get mixed with items, or with another mother's breast milk.

❖ Only thaw/warm milk needed at any given feeding. Do not thaw/warm milk in advance to save time, because the milk could be wasted.

Finally, slowly introduce your child to his new setting. Don't just drop him off on your first day back to work. Your breastfed baby is used to tender loving care, and will need to warm up to his new caregiver. Start by taking your baby with you to your initial child-care provider visits. Once you think you've made a decision, take him for one or two hours while you are there with him. This will show him that the environment is one that you approve of. Then, take him and leave him there for one or two hours without you. See how he handles it. The next time, leave him for four hours. Next time, for six hours. Test the waters. See if it's a good fit for him. Remember to say good-bye to the baby when you leave. It's tempting to sneak off to ward off a crying confrontation. This is a trap and can make things worse. It's best for him to see you leave and not look up expecting to find you, and becoming shocked to see you are nowhere in sight. Ask the staff member who cares for him how he did during that time, if he cried often, if they were able to settle him down.

By testing this new routine, you'll also be able to see different aspects of the child care setting, since you'll be popping in and out. This does not mean spy on them, but you need to see the setting from all angles, and not just the one presented to you during your initial visit. Watch for the attitudes of the staff, and the cleanliness of the site at different times of the day. Are things consistent? If your baby seems completely out of sorts, or if your instinct says, "something isn't right," then follow your gut. There's a saying, "doubt means don't do." Your intuition is powerful and is always right. Feel free to go with that feeling with confidence. And if you allow enough time for interviewing and practicing, you'll find a child-care provider that is not only breastfeeding friendly, but one who will be a good addition to your extended family.

Chapter Seven

The Truth about Breastfeeding Myths

A myth is a belief that is not true, but is thought to be factual or partly true. We read of myths about the Greek gods, the Tooth Fairy, vampires, and even "hiccups mean you're growing." Myths have little or no scientific basis. Although we believe them to be true, they are not. Some myths are fun and harmless. The Tooth Fairy, for instance, is a mythical figure; yet millions of children around the country place their lost teeth under the pillow at night expecting a treat in the morning in exchange for the tooth. Other myths are potentially dangerous.

Breastfeeding myths have thoroughly saturated our community. Belief in these myths has caused many African American women to not even consider breastfeeding. Because so few of us are breastfeeding, our babies die more than others, and have more health problems that last far into childhood. You may have heard some of these myths. You may even believe them to be true. Read on, and let's dissect them to find the truth about the following breastfeeding myths that have discouraged many of our women from breastfeeding.

"Breastfeeding is disgusting!"

This is the mantra of many young women across the country today, especially pregnant teens. Breastfeeding is not disgusting, but is a natural way to feed our babies. The problem is that we are disconnected from what our bodies are designed to do, and the term "natural" is not appealing to everyone. The root of this myth is twofold: the way we view our bodies, and the lack of African American breastfeeding role models.

It doesn't take long to see that our country is very image-conscious. We're very much focused on our physical appearance. Our bodies are used to sell everything. Take a look at TV commercials. Advertisements for all sorts of products use the body as a sex symbol to sell the product. Ads for underclothes, not long ago, didn't show the whole woman's body. Now, men and women are seen full length to sell underwear. The body is used to sell cologne, food, medication, and household appliances.

The body as a sex symbol is also exploited on TV shows. Nudity on regular TV stations has increased tenfold over the past ten years. Now it's not unusual to see someone's rear end in the shower, or the silhouette of the whole naked body behind a shower curtain. And that's just regular TV. Cable television has gone above and beyond in the area of body and sex exposure.

Music videos have also contributed significantly to the exposure of our bodies in public. More than half of the videos today exhibit women in scantily clad outfits with most body parts exposed, leaving little room for imagination. The women dance provocatively. There is no subtlety here. Ironically, the object of these music videos, commercials, advertisements, and TV shows are women. Our bodies are being exploited and exposed, making us objects of sexuality, and little else. Yes, we are sexual beings, yet that's a far cry from the way our bodies are abused. We don't see men naked, or almost naked in music videos or selling products. In fact, in most music videos, men wear layers upon layers of clothes. Sadly, most people don't recognize this exploitation of women. We watch the music videos and buy the clothes that give the world a view of our most private places. Movies depict us in sexual acts, often violent.

African American women particularly have a narrow image in the media, and are often viewed as sex objects. In rap videos, we are portrayed as sex goddesses, wearing skimpy, all too revealing clothes. Our often shapely forms are glorified for physical appeal, and not for our inner beauty or intellect. This is not to say that women need to be covered from head to toe, but the music videos send the wrong message about African American women. It makes us objects of desire, instead of intelligent and valuable members of society.

Other stereotypical images of African American women are that of the super career-seeker, neck-twisting "I gotta get mine," or the all-too-familiar mammy. The career type is often shown as having little time for family, and on upwardly mobile track career advancement, regardless of family obligations—like children. She feels, the media would have you believe, that making money is far more important than caring for a family. If she has a husband and children, she buries herself in her work.

The neck-twisting sistah is always sashaying around with her hands on her hips and a smirk on her face. She always has an attitude, and is often shown cutting her African American man down to size. She generally has two or more kids, by different men, and is a single mother. She wears clothes that are tight and formfitting.

The historical type is the mammy, a demeaning caricature of the African American woman. We've seen her as the Aunt Jemima figure, capable in the kitchen, able to clean house and watch either the master's children or upper class white families, all the while smiling and happy to care for them. She often had to neglect her own children and family. Ironically, this harmful image was used in the early 1900s by department stores to advertise merchandise.

So, what does this have to do with breastfeeding? It's all about how our bodies are viewed. As you can see, breasts are 99 percent of the time only referred to in media and popular culture in sexual terms. Breasts are for the purpose of sexual pleasure or advertising merchandise, if you believe what you see on TV, in movies, or in many print publications. The other 1 percent of the time, breasts are discussed in medical terms—for breast cancer prevention campaigns or surgery. Rarely are breasts discussed with breastfeeding. In fact, you only hear about breast milk on TV shows as a substance that "you don't want to mistake for regular milk" in the fridge; or occasionally, breastfeeding supporters get a shot at mentioning breastfeeding on a news show or in an article. Unfortunately, these instances are few.

As a result, few women, as seen by the low breastfeeding rates in this country—especially that of African American women—have the opportunity to hear breasts discussed in a positive light. Many of us have bought into the image of breasts as a symbol of sex. We look at our own breasts and size them up against other women. Where once getting breast implants was something for the rich, you can now buy them on a payment plan. We don't look at our breasts as a means to nourish and nurture our babies.

Women of all ages, who do not know who they are (unsure of their purpose in life and worth as a woman), who have low self-esteem, or who have suffered mental and/or sexual abuse receive these messages unconsciously. These images sexualize our breasts in our minds, then when breastfeeding enters the picture, we instantly frown and look disgusted. We deliver birth to multiple children, but work hard to get rid of the milk that naturally fills our breasts within days of childbirth. Unfortunately, many African American babies become ill, and even die because we have a negative image about our breasts and what they are designed for.

"Breastfeeding hurts."

Let's be clear right up front: Breastfeeding should not hurt! It is designed so well that, when done properly, it should not hurt. Just as your body and all its organs have the ability to maintain your health while a baby is growing inside of you, so your breasts are prepared to provide nourishment for your baby—even when he has a full set of teeth.

When someone has a bad experience, she tends to share that information with friends. Unfortunately, when African American women have bad breastfeeding experiences, it runs deeper than sharing that experience with friends. We share that information with family, friends, coworkers, anyone who'll listen, it seems. This belief that breastfeeding is painful has left a stigma with us for generations.

The key point to remember here is that breastfeeding shouldn't hurt if done the right way. Let's look at why breastfeeding shouldn't hurt. As breastfeeding is a learning experience for both you and your baby, keep in mind that there may be some discomfort during the first few weeks. Take heart that once you understand how breastfeeding works, you'll have a pain-free experience.

The best way to understand how this works is to look at your breasts in the mirror. It's important for you to become familiar with them. You will notice that there is a darker area around your nipple, which is the areola. This is the area that should be the target for your baby's mouth: Not your nipple. The nipple is more delicate than the areola, and that's not where the milk is. The milk is stored behind or under your areola. Your baby needs to have his mouth target that darker area, because this is where he will be able to get your breast milk. By compressing his gums onto your areola, your baby triggers the milk sinuses beneath that release the nutritional breast milk they're holding.

If your baby latches onto your nipple, it will hurt, and you may become discouraged. This is understandable. After hours of labor and delivery, who wants any more pain, right? Your body is so wonderfully made that it's giving you a cue that something isn't going right with breastfeeding. Also, when your baby is latched onto your nipple instead of your areola, he will not get all of the breast milk that he needs to grow because the milk is not stored in the nipple and he may not be able to stimulate the letdown of your milk, potentially causing engorgement. However, when your baby is latched onto your areola, your nipple will be pulled towards the back roof of his mouth, which is a soft, safe area for your nipple to be while breastfeeding. Remember: your baby's mouth is small, so it won't take much for your nipple to get in that space.

If you're in pain while breastfeeding, chances are the baby is not latched on the right way, or is not positioned properly. Let's briefly look at positioning, which is more fully covered in chapter 2. You hold your baby's body in a straight line by holding him close and being sure that his stomach flat against yours and his head is facing your breast. This keeps his neck in a straight line so that when he's nursing, he will maintain a good latch, and can swallow effectively. If his body is slanted or tilted, if his stomach is leaning away from yours, then it will cause his body weight to pull his head away from your breast, even while he's latched on. This can cause you nipple pain and/or damage. Also, when he's not positioned well, he won't be able to swallow the amount that he needs to grow.

You need to be positioned properly as well. If you're not comfortable, then you can make your breastfeeding experience even more difficult. Try to sit in your favorite chair or lie down, which should give you full use of your hands, and access to your baby. Prop a pillow behind your head or back, or under your feet. You can also use a pillow to help you to support the baby, or to place across your stomach if you had a c-section. If it helps, put your feet up on an ottoman or stack of pillows. Whatever it takes to make you feel comfortable, do it.

If you continue to feel pain even after you're sure the baby's latched properly, then you should investigate whether you have thrush or another problem that can be solved with prompt medical attention (see chapter 2).

So, does breastfeeding hurt? Absolutely not, if it's done properly with a good latch and good positioning. If you maintain your commitment to breastfeed, then you'll have much greater success. Tell yourself, "I can do this. I can do this. If I feel pain, then I have a clue that something isn't quite right. I can start over and try again. I can do this." Your healthy baby will be the result of this mantra.

"Breast milk is not enough to feed a baby."

This myth is based largely on the fact that you can't measure how much breast milk a baby is receiving. Breast milk is full of just the right amount of fat, vitamins, minerals, and other important nutrients your baby needs for optimal growth and health. In fact, breast milk is all your baby needs— no food, no water, no other supplement—for the first six months of life! It even changes with the growing nutritional needs of your baby. For instance, if you notice that your baby is eating more frequently, then he's probably going through a growth spurt. His extra nursing is helping your body to bring the quantity and nutritional value up to meet his growth needs. That's amazing!

The belief that breast milk is insufficient for a baby is based on the following misconceptions we have about babies:

- ❖ If a breastfed baby drinks a bottle of formula after a feeding at the breast, he is still hungry.
- ❖ A happy baby does not cry.
- ❖ Breastfed babies eat all the time and never seem satisfied.

Before we dig too deeply into this myth, it's important to look at the culture of African Americans and our relationship with food. In Africa, we enjoyed bountiful and healthy foods, and obesity was not an issue. Except in times of famine, our eating habits were healthy.

The impact of slavery in our history greatly altered our diet and dietary habits. During slavery, we had to learn a new way of preparing food. The very selection of foods in this country was foreign to us. The slave diet consisted primarily of pork, cornmeal, and molasses. This forced a change in our nutritional practices, and our view of food. Food was once abundant in Africa, with little fear of hunger, or only temporary seasons of hunger. Once in America, food was scarce. As slaves, we were generally given foods in rations, which consisted of pork (high in fat) and cornmeal—high in sugar content, which ultimately breaks down into fat.

This is obviously not an optimal diet for healthy living. Slowly, our view of food changed. We had to become ingenious to manage the unique food, and the sparseness of it. Foods high in fat, pork for instance, became a staple in our diet. This was a shock to our systems because previously, high-fat food was rare. High-fat foods, in abundance, over a long period of time, began to change our state of health. Overindulgent eating, or binging, was introduced into our culture out of a necessity to eat in abundance when food was available, and to bulk up our bodies with fat to cope with cold weather conditions.

Today, the African American diet is still largely unhealthy, which is evident in our deadly rates of hypertension, obesity, diabetes, and other diseases. It is not uncommon to find well-meaning mothers, grandmothers, and aunties across the country feeding infants under two months of age anything from rice cereal, mashed potatoes, bananas, and applesauce, among other things. Bottled breast milk and infant formula is often padded with rice or oat cereal. This is done as early as four weeks, based on a belief that it will help the baby have a full stomach and thus sleep longer. A plump, round-faced baby is a happy baby. This is probably associated with distant imprints in our brain of slave times when our babies often died from malnutrition and starvation.

When you give a baby a bottle of infant formula, you can measure the amount the baby will receive. You can visualize that the baby will consume any number of ounces at a given feeding. You fill the bottle with formula, water, juice, whatever, and you can almost see the baby's stomach being filled with that form of nourishment. When a baby is breastfed, you simply can't see the volume of milk the baby is receiving. This is a cause of concern for many African American women. Counting diapers and monitoring weight gain is rarely enough to calm our fear of our babies starving. This is especially true if a baby is born with a low birth weight, which is more normal than not in our community. Let's look back at those misconceptions.

"If a breastfed baby drinks a bottle of formula after a feeding at the breast, he is still hungry."

Breast milk is easily digested, which is why infants need to breastfeed often, at least every two hours in the beginning. When a baby breastfeeds, the nutrients in breast milk become readily available for the baby. So, all of the nutrients the baby needs goes to all the right places. And since breast milk is designed specifically for an infant's stomach, it is tolerated well and digested quickly; unlike infant formula, which lingers in your baby's system, often causing diarrhea, constipation, or other stomach upset. It would follow, then, that even after being breastfed, a growing baby, if offered, may drink a bottle of infant formula. This does not mean that the breast milk was insufficient.

"Breastfed babies eat all the time, and never seem satisfied."

Breastfeeding does not just serve the purpose of nourishment. It also soothes a baby's need to suckle. Babies have a strong sucking reflex from their time in the womb, and it increases intensely after birth. You can see sonogram pictures of babies with a thumb or hand in their mouth, while in the mom's uterus. Many women use pacifiers to provide that sucking relief for their baby. Have you ever noticed that many babies use pacifiers, and continue to use them well in their toddler years? What better way to provide that stimulation and release than at the breast?

"Breastfeeding makes your breasts sag!"

A woman's breasts are set on a course of change from early adolescence, beginning as early as age nine, sometimes earlier. When a young girl's breasts begin to "bud," the cells in her breasts start preparation for continued growth. During puberty, her breasts will continue to change and grow in shape and size, with continued cell development for eventual pregnancy. Through a woman's childbearing years, her breasts will be in a constant state of change. If she gains or loses weight, she'll notice a change in her breasts' shape, size, and level of gravity. Her breasts may sag before pregnancy, much less from breastfeeding. When a woman becomes pregnant, her breast tissues and cells prepare for breastfeeding, creating all that's needed to provide milk for her baby. Her breasts will often double their size during her prenatal period. During her breastfeeding experience, her breasts will initially grow during the early days. Then they'll level off for a time, and often will get smaller, or return to their prepregnancy size after breastfeeding ends.

Are breastfeeding women the only ones whose breasts sag? Of course not! The lingerie industry is booming because of the various bras designed to provide that lift so many women desire. Yet, breastfeeding rates, in general, are low. This means that women are suffering from sagging breasts, regardless of their choice to breastfeed or not.

Another factor influencing sagging breasts is genetics. If a woman is shaped like her mother or grandmother who has sagging breasts, chances are, she'll have them, too. If a woman does not work out and stay fit, her breasts are also likely to sag. There are also many women who never become pregnant who have sagging breasts as well. This might be due to genetics, weight gain/loss, or some other factor.

"Breastfeeding means I'll never be free."

Most breastfeeding educators are known for teaching how convenient breastfeeding is. Breast milk is always ready and always the right temperature. You never have to worry about milk spoiling or warming bottles. Running out of milk is never a problem. You can actually get more rest while breastfeeding because you can do it lying down, and because it creates a hormone that actually relaxes you. Dad even gets more rest because he doesn't have to get up to make bottles in the middle of the night. You can even run out of the house on an errand without a diaper bag; just stick a diaper and some wipes in your purse, and you and baby are ready to go. Sounds pretty convenient, right?

Not for a number of us, especially young African American mothers. Many African American women feel that those areas of convenience do more to tie them down than anything else. They feel that they will never be free of their baby or the "job" of breastfeeding. They believe that by breastfeeding, they'll be tied down to the home and the baby, and won't be able to go out and live their lives. They would rather give up optimal health for their baby and themselves than breastfeed, so they can go back to previous activities.

For the teen mother, this belief in breastfeeding as a lack of freedom is difficult to overcome. She already feels the pressure of being a teen mother, with many of her previous liberties on the brink of extinction because she has someone else to care for. The woman between age twenty and thirty often feels that breastfeeding will hinder her ability to pursue her career or educational opportunities. Both types of women equate breastfeeding with being tied down.

The truth is, whether a woman breastfeeds or not, she'll have to spend the bulk of her time for the next eighteen or more years caring for the health and welfare of her child. A baby needs to be attached to his mother. Attachment is not negative. A baby needs to be held, kissed, loved! A baby needs physical contact to let him know he's safe and secure. There is no such thing as spoiling a baby. Other words for spoil are: mess up, ruin, and destroy. How is loving, feeding, and caring for a baby's needs messing him up, ruining, or destroying him? On the contrary, babies who feel secure will thrive.

Freedom is really a state of mind. There seems to be a disconnection between women and their babies these days. Everyone wants the baby to quickly sleep through the night, hold his own bottle, and begin walking! Babies are no longer allowed to grow naturally, on their own terms. Mothers are in a rush to get baby used to the bottle so she can get out and be free. There is no question that peace of mind and quiet time for your own thoughts are key for you to remain mentally and emotionally healthy to care for your family. However, your baby must be your priority. When you become pregnant, it does not mean that your life is over, it just means life is now different. Remember, your baby did not ask to be born, and it's your responsibility as a mother to care for that baby's every need. So, freedom, to a certain extent, will be halted for a moment, but not taken away all together.

Breastfeeding actually provides greater freedom for you because you're freed up from the tasks of bottle-feeding and worrying about your baby's health. Breastfeeding actually builds confidence in women (see chapter 9) and their babies. Breastfeeding gives you peace of mind that your baby is happy and healthy, affording you mental freedom, which can take you far.

"I can't breastfeed…I have to go back to work."

Just as "location, location, location" is important in the success of a business, so is "information, information, information" important in the area of shattering breastfeeding myths. Many of us say, "Oh, I'll breastfeed while I'm home, but I have to stop when I go back to work." There is a general lack of knowledge about breast pumps in our community. Since we receive such minimal information about breastfeeding during our prenatal period, we don't learn about the different pumps on the market.

Most employers are reluctant to give any extra time for maternity, much less provide a breastfeeding room for their staff. Women who work in restaurants, retail stores, or blue-collar jobs are concerned about finding a private place to pump milk.

You can return to work and continue to breastfeed, successfully. See chapter 5. It's important that you do so for your baby's health, and your own.

"I will have to stop eating the foods I like if I breast-feed, especially spicy food."

No, you won't. There are absolutely no foods you can't eat. You can continue to eat your regular diet and all the foods you enjoy. By eating a wide variety of foods from all the food groups, you are allowing your baby to experience different tastes. Breast milk actually takes on the flavor of the foods you eat. Not the exact same flavor you taste, but a hint of the flavor, including the spices you eat.

Do Mexican, Indian, Caribbean, or Asian women not breastfeed? Their diets are full of a variety of spices, with varying degrees of heat. They still breastfeed their babies. In fact, since their diets are rich in spices helps to prepare their babies to be better able to tolerate their culture's dietary practices.

Cabbage, onions, broccoli, garlic, and milk have all received a bad reputation of being unacceptable foods to eat if you're breastfeeding. This is simply not so. You can eat absolutely anything you want, including junk food. You can also drink caffeine while breastfeeding. The key factor here is being in tune with your baby. If you notice that your baby is particularly uncomfortable every time you eat a certain food, then you can be reasonably sure that that particular food doesn't sit well with your baby's stomach. You don't have to radically change your diet. You can still eat the foods you enjoy, with a bit of moderation where necessary, like with caffeine. Breastfeeding is not about what you can't have, but more about eating in a way that will allow you to be healthy and refueled for your breastfeeding experience.

There are two simple precautions you should take in your diet. One, you need to be sure that you are eating a well-balanced diet, based on the food guide pyramid. Moderation is key to maintaining a healthy lifestyle. Exercising at least three days a week for thirty to forty-five minutes or more is also recommended by many physicians and personal trainers across the country. It's important for you to eat well because your baby is taking many of your nutritional stores; what's left over belongs to you. So, if you're eating well, then you can maintain good health throughout your breastfeeding experience.

Second, if you have a history of food allergies, be it dairy, wheat, shellfish, etc., then there may be a chance that your baby has that same sensitivity to a particular food. For example, if a woman is allergic to dairy or is lactose intolerant, and eats a dairy product, she may notice that her baby becomes ill during those times. This may mean that her baby is allergic to dairy products. On the other hand, she may be allergic to dairy, but her baby may not respond negatively to his mother eating it. The key factor here is to know your history, know your food sensitivities, and then watch your baby. He will let you know if he can't tolerate a particular food.

Other than those precautions, eat, drink, and be merry throughout your breastfeeding experience—be it a few months, or better yet, a few years.

"Formula is just as good as breast milk!"

Infant formula is an inferior, substandard, low-grade, second-rate alternative to breast milk.

Many African Americans, both men and women, are under the false belief that infant formula is just as good as breast milk. They say, "Formula has all the vitamins, minerals, and nutrients a baby needs." That's exactly what infant formula companies would have you believe. There are some significant differences between breast milk and infant formula that are worth looking at. Keep in mind that breast milk is as old as humankind, while infant formula is just about one hundred years old.

All pregnant women and dads-to-be learn early on that babies should not be given cow's milk before their first birthday. The primary reason is that babies can't sufficiently digest the minerals and proteins in cow's milk. The secondary reason is that cow's milk is made for calves, not for infants. The nutrients made up of cow's milk are deficient in most of the vitamins, minerals, and fatty acids that a human infant needs to survive. Cow's milk is made for the growth of a cow, which is at least two to three times faster than infants. It's made to grow a calf into a full-grown cow, with limited intelligence, not for the growth and brain development of the most intelligent species on the planet: humans. The opposite is also true. The content of human breast milk would not be sufficient for the growth of a calf into an adult cow. The same is true of cow's milk for human infants.

The main ingredient in infant formula is cow's milk. Infant formula is just that—a scientific equation or recipe. The following is a list of ingredients found in the typical can of premixed infant formula: cow's milk (which includes butterfat, whey, lactose), palm olein oil, soy oil, coconut oil, high oleic sunflower oil, omon and diglycerides, soy lecithin, carrageenan, vitamin A palmitate, vitamin D3, vitamin E acetate, vitamin K1, thiamin hydrochloride, pantothenate, biotin, sodium ascorbate, ascorbic acid, inositol, calcium chloride, calcium phosphate, ferrous sulfate, zinc sulfate, manganese sulfate, cupric sulfate, sodium chloride, sodium citrate, potassium citrate, potassium hydroxide, sodium selenate, taurin, and nucleotides. If you can't pronounce it, do you want to give it to your infant?

Besides knowing that infant formula is created in a scientific laboratory and manufacturing plant using genetically engineered ingredients, you should also know a few other key differences about breast milk and infant formula.

First, infant formula does not provide your baby any protection from any germ, illness, or disease. Your infant is thrust from the safety of your womb into a germ-infested world. He'll need the protection that only your breast milk can provide. Infant formula, with all of its ingredients, cannot protect your baby from the following potentially deadly illnesses: colds, ear infections, sudden infant death syndrome, diarrhea/constipation, childhood diabetes, obesity, asthma, allergies, pneumonia, and upper respiratory infections. Your new baby is at risk for all of the above—especially African American babies, who have some of the highest risks of infant death, asthma, and obesity.

If you don't give him breast milk, you are leaving him vulnerable to illnesses that could be lifelong, or life-threatening. Even the potential of dealing with a sick baby should be enough to take all consideration about using infant formula out of your mind. Babies fed infant formula are sick more often, require more hospitalization, and cost the government millions of dollars in health care costs, from medications, surgery, and other fees associated with being sick.

Second, infant formula does not provide the optimal balance of nutrients for your baby's brain development. Think about it. Why would you give your baby a product that is biologically designed for the brain development of a cow? Can a cow ever compete mentally or physically with a human? Can a cow use reason or common sense? Can a cow know whether to cross the street at a red light, balance a checkbook, apologize, cook a meal, or attend school? No, a cow could not do any of the above. In fact, a cow's life generally consists of grazing in pastures and moving at a slow, leisurely pace—not exactly the most favorable brain food for the advancement of society, is it?

Your newborn needs food from the start, which will be the basis for expanding and growing his brain. Studies have even shown that breastfed babies have higher IQs (i.e., intellect and brain power and ability) than babies who are fed infant formula. Since African Americans tend to have a more difficult life than other races, wouldn't you want to provide a jump start that could make a difference throughout his entire life? Why not give him your breast milk, which can give him a head start in a life that is often plagued with social stereotypes and institutional harassment?

Third, infant formula does not help to develop your baby's eye coordination, or promote strong dental health. Have you ever seen a picture of a baby with baby bottle tooth decay (BBTD)? In extreme cases, the gums turn black and the teeth are rotted. It's an uncomfortable existence for a baby, and it also forces a baby to begin the often painful process of advanced dental work.

Fourth, infant formula does not provide any benefits or protection for you! Infant formula does not:

- ❖ Help your uterus to go back to a normal, healthy size, or prevent afterbirth hemorrhaging.
- ❖ Burn up to one thousand calories a day the way breast milk does.
- ❖ Protect you from ovarian cancer, premenopausal breast cancer, or osteoporosis.
- ❖ Give you more rest.
- ❖ Create hormones that make you love and bond with your baby.
- ❖ Delay ovulation or protect you from pregnancy.
- ❖ Save you money!
- ❖ Reduce the time you may have to take off from work to care for a sick baby.
- ❖ Improve your self-esteem.

Fifth, infant formula is not environmentally safe. Infant formula is a 2 billion-dollar-a-year industry, so you can imagine the amount of waste going into the earth—waste that can harm the earth, such as aluminum from formula cans, plastic from bottles and bottle liners, rubber from artificial nipples, and paper from infant formula advertisements in newspapers, magazines, and brochures. If you don't recycle, and millions of people across the country don't, these items can damage the earth further.

Ultimately, the choice is yours. Only you can provide the best, most advantageous start to your baby's life. Give the best to your African American baby, and reap the benefits for you, your baby, and society!

However, there are instances where women—for reasons from low milk supply to maternal or infant health issues—can't breastfeed their babies. In these cases, infant formula, whether milk or soy-based, can be safely used.

"No one is breastfeeding anymore."

This myth has some truth because the breastfeeding rates of African American women are lower than most other races. However, the ones that do breastfeed tend to be more private with it. They are less likely to breastfeed in public—even around friends and family.

More Breastfeeding Myths and Facts from Dr. Jack Newman, renowned lactation expert
Reprinted with permission

"Nursing mothers cannot breastfeed if they have had X-rays."

Not true! Regular X-rays, such as a chest X-ray or dental X-ray, do not affect the milk or the baby, and the mother may nurse without concern. Mammograms are harder to read when the mother is lactating, but can be done, and the mother should not stop breastfeeding just to get this done. There are other ways of investigating a breast lump. Newer imaging methods such as CT scans and MRI scans are of no concern, even if contrast is used. And special X-rays using contrast media? As long as no radioactive isotope is used, there is no concern, and the mother should not stop even for one feeding.

However, as we often do these very same tests on children, even small babies, and the potential loss of benefits if the mother stops breastfeeding are considerable, the mother should continue breastfeeding. The exception is the thyroid scan. This test must be avoided in breastfeeding mothers. There are many ways of evaluating the thyroid, and only very occasionally does a thyroid scan truly have to be done. Check first before taking the radioactive iodine—the test can wait until you know for sure. In many cases where the scan must be done, it can be put off for several months.

"Breastfeeding mothers' milk can 'dry up' just like that."

Not true! If this can occur, it must be a rare occurrence. Aside from day to day and morning to evening variations, milk production does not change suddenly. There are changes that occur that may make it seem as if milk production is suddenly much less: an increase in the needs of the baby (the so-called growth spurt is the most common). If this is the reason for the seemingly insufficient milk, a few days of more frequent nursing will bring things back to normal. Try compressing the breast with your hand to help the baby get more milk.

At about five to six weeks of age, more or less, babies who would fall asleep at the breast when the flow of milk slowed down tend to start pulling at the breast or crying when the milk flow slows. The milk has not dried up, but the baby has changed. Try compressing the breast with your hand to help the baby get more milk.

The mother's breasts do not seem full or are soft.

It is normal after a few weeks for the mother no longer to have engorgement, or even fullness of the breasts. As long as the baby is drinking at the breast, do not be concerned.

The baby breastfeeds less well.

This is often due to the baby being given bottles or pacifiers, and thus, learning an inappropriate way of breastfeeding.

The birth control pill may decrease your milk supply.

Think about stopping the pill, or changing to a progesterone-only pill. Or use other methods of birth control. If the baby truly seems not to be getting enough, get help, but do not introduce a bottle, which will only make things worse. If absolutely necessary, the baby can be supplemented by using a lactation aid that will not interfere with breastfeeding. However, lots can be done before taking supplements. Get help.

"Physicians know a lot about breastfeeding."

Not true! Obviously, there are exceptions. However, very few physicians trained in North America or Western Europe learned anything at all about breastfeeding in medical school. Even fewer learned about the practical aspects of helping mothers start breastfeeding, and helping them maintain breastfeeding. After medical school, most of the information physicians get regarding infant feeding comes from formula company representatives or advertisements.

"Pediatricians, at least, know a lot about breastfeeding."

Not true! Obviously, there are exceptions. However, in their post-medical school training (residency), most pediatricians learned nothing formal about breastfeeding, and what they picked up in passing was often wrong. To many trainees in pediatrics, breastfeeding is seen as an "obstacle to the good medical care" of hospitalized babies.

"Formula company literature and free formula samples do not influence whether, or how long, a mother breastfeeds."

Really? So why do the formula companies work so hard to make sure that new mothers are given their company's samples? Are these samples and the literature given out to encourage breastfeeding? Is the cost of the samples and booklets taken on by formula companies so that mothers will be encouraged to breastfeed longer? The companies often argue that if the mother does give formula, they want the mother to use their brand. In competing with each other, the formula companies also compete with breastfeeding. Did you believe that argument when the cigarette companies used it?

"Breast milk given with formula may cause problems for the baby."

Not true! Most breastfeeding mothers do not need to use formula; and when problems arise that seem to require artificial milk, often the problems can be resolved without resorting to formula. However, when the baby may require formula, there is no reason that breast milk and formula cannot be given together.

"Babies who are breastfed on demand are likely to be 'colicky.'"

Not true! "Colicky" breastfed babies often gain weight very quickly, and sometimes are feeding frequently. However, many are colicky not because they are feeding frequently, but because they do not take the high-fat milk as well as they should. Typically, the baby drinks very well for the first few minutes, then nibbles or sleeps. When the baby is offered the other side, he will drink well again for a short while and then nibble or sleep. The baby will fill up with relatively low-fat milk, and thus feed frequently. The taking in of mostly low-fat milk may also result in gas, crying, and explosive watery bowel movements. The mother can urge the baby to breastfeed longer on the first side, and thus get more higher-fat milk, by compressing the breast once the baby no longer actually swallows at the breast.

"Mothers who receive immunizations (tetanus, rubella, hepatitis B, hepatitis A, etc.) should stop breastfeeding for twenty-four hours (or three days, or two weeks)."

Not true! Why should they? There is no risk for the baby, and he may even benefit. The rare exception is the baby who has an immune deficiency. In that case, the mother should not receive an immunization with a weakened live virus (e.g., oral, but not injectable polio, or measles, mumps, rubella) even if the baby is being fed artificially.

"There is no such thing as nipple confusion."

Not true! A baby who is only bottle-fed for the first two weeks of life, for example, will usually refuse to take the breast, even if the mother has an abundant supply. A baby who has had the breast only for three or four months is unlikely to take the bottle. Some babies prefer the right or left breast to the other. Bottle-fed babies often prefer one artificial nipple to another. So there is such a thing as preferring one nipple to another. The only question is how quickly it can occur. Given the right set of circumstances, the preference can occur after one or two bottles. The baby, having difficulties latching on, may never have had an artificial nipple, but the introduction of an artificial nipple rarely improves the situation, and often makes it much worse. Note that many who say there is no such thing as nipple confusion also advise the mother to start a bottle early so that the baby will not refuse it.

"Women with flat or inverted nipples cannot breastfeed."

Not true! Babies do not breastfeed on nipples, they breastfeed on the breast. Though it may be easier for a baby to latch onto a breast with a prominent nipple, it is not necessary for nipples to stick out. A proper start will usually prevent problems, and mothers with any-shaped nipples can breastfeed perfectly adequately. In the past, a nipple shield was frequently suggested to get the baby to take the breast. This gadget should not be used, especially in the first few days! Though it may seem a solution, its use often results in poor feeding and severe weight loss, and makes it even more difficult to get the baby to take the breast. If the baby does not take the breast at first with proper help, he will often take the breast later. Breasts also change in the first few weeks, and as long as the mother maintains a good milk supply, the baby will usually latch on, sooner or later.

"A woman who becomes pregnant must stop breastfeeding."

Not true! If the mother and child desire, breastfeeding can continue. There are women who continue nursing the older child even after delivery of the new baby. Many women do decide to stop nursing when they become pregnant because their nipples are sore, or for other reasons, but there is no rush or medical necessity to do so. In fact, there are often good reasons to continue. The milk supply may decrease during pregnancy, but if the baby is taking other foods, this is not a problem.

"A baby with diarrhea should not breastfeed."

Not true! The best treatment for a gut infection (gastroenteritis) is breastfeeding. Furthermore, it is very unusual for the baby to require fluids other than breast milk. If lactose intolerance, which causes diarrhea and gastro upset, is a problem, the baby can receive lactase drops (available without prescription) just before or after the feeding, but this is rarely necessary in breastfeeding babies. Get information on its use from the clinic. In any case, lactose intolerance due to gastroenteritis will disappear with time. Lactose-free formula is not better than breastfeeding. Breastfeeding is better than any formula.

"Babies will stay on the breast for two hours because they like to suck."

Not true! Babies need and like to suck, but how much do they need? Most babies who stay at the breast for such a long time are probably hungry, even though they may be gaining well. Being at the breast is not the same as drinking at the breast. Latching the baby better onto the breast allows the baby to nurse more effectively, and thus spend more time actually drinking. You can also help the baby to drink more by expressing milk into his mouth when he no longer swallows on his own. Babies younger than five to six weeks often fall asleep at the breast because the flow of milk is slow, not necessarily because they have had enough to eat.

"Babies need to know how to take a bottle, so a bottle should always be introduced before the baby refuses to take one."

Not true! Though many mothers decide to introduce a bottle for various reasons, there is no reason a baby must learn how to use one. Indeed, there is no great advantage in a baby's taking a bottle. Since Canadian women are supposed to receive twenty-six weeks maternity leave, the baby can be started eating solids before the mother goes back to her outside work. The baby can even take fluids or solids that are quite liquid-y off a spoon. At about six months of age, the baby can start learning how to drink from a cup, and though it may take several weeks for him to learn to use it efficiently, he will learn.

If the mother is going to introduce a bottle, it is better if she waits until the baby has been nursing well for four to six weeks, and then only give it occasionally. Sometimes, however, babies who take the bottle well at six weeks refuse it at three or four months, even if they have been getting bottles regularly (smart babies). Do not worry, and proceed as above with solids and spoon. Giving a bottle when breastfeeding is going badly is not a good idea and usually makes the breastfeeding even more difficult. For your sake and the baby's, do not try to "starve the baby into submission." Get help.

"If a mother has surgery, she has to wait a day before restarting nursing."

Not true! The mother can breastfeed immediately after surgery, as soon as she is up to it. Neither the medications used during anesthesia nor pain medications, nor antibiotics used after surgery require the mother to avoid breastfeeding, except under exceptional circumstances. Enlightened hospitals will accommodate breastfeeding mothers and babies when either one needs to be admitted to the hospital, so that breastfeeding can continue. Many rules that restrict breastfeeding are more for the convenience of staff than for the benefit of mothers and babies.

"Breastfeeding twins is too difficult to manage."

Not true! If breastfeeding is going well, it is easier than bottle-feeding twins. This is why it is so important that a special effort should be made to get breastfeeding started right when the mother has had twins. Many women have breastfed triplets exclusively. This obviously takes a lot of work and time, but twins and triplets take a lot of work and time no matter how the infants are fed.

"Women whose breasts do not enlarge, or enlarge only a little during pregnancy, will not produce enough milk."

Not true! There are a very few women who cannot produce enough milk (though they can continue to breastfeed by supplementing with a lactation aid). Some of these women say that their breasts did not enlarge during pregnancy. However, the vast majority of women whose breasts do not seem to enlarge during pregnancy produce more than enough milk.

"If a mother's breasts do not seem full, they have little milk in them."

Not true! Breasts do not have to feel full to produce plenty of milk. It is normal that a breastfeeding woman's breasts feel less full as her body adjusts to her baby's milk intake. This can happen suddenly, and may occur as early as two weeks after birth, or even earlier. The breast is never "empty," and even produces milk as the baby nurses.

"Breastfeeding in public is not decent."

Not true! It is the humiliation and harassment of mothers who are nursing their babies that is not decent. Women who are trying to do the best for their babies should not be forced by other people's lack of understanding to stay home or feed their babies in public washrooms. Those who are offended need only to avert their eyes. Children will not be damaged psychologically by seeing a women breastfeeding. On the contrary, they might learn something important, beautiful, and fascinating. They might even learn that breasts are not only for selling beer. Other women who have left their babies at home to be bottle-fed while they went out might be encouraged to bring the baby with them the next time.

"Breastfeeding a child until three or four years of age is abnormal and bad for the child, causing an over-dependent relationship between mother and child."

Not true! Breastfeeding for two to four years was the rule in most cultures since the beginning of time. Only in the last one hundred years or so has breastfeeding been seen as something to be limited. Children nursed into the third year are not overly dependent. On the contrary, they tend to be very secure, and thus, more independent. They themselves will make the step to stop breastfeeding (sometimes with gentle encouragement from the mother), and will be secure in their accomplishment.

"If the baby is off the breast for a few days (or weeks), the mother should not restart breastfeeding because the milk sours."

Not true! The milk is as good as it ever was. Milk in the breast is not milk or formula in a bottle.

"After exercise a mother should not breastfeed."

Not true! There is absolutely no reason why a mother would not be able to breastfeed after exercising. The study that purported to show that babies were fussy when feeding after mother exercises was poorly done and contradicts the everyday experience of millions of mothers.

"Breastfeeding is blamed for everything."

True! Family, health professionals, neighbors, friends, and taxi drivers will blame breastfeeding if the mother is tired, nervous, weepy, sick, has pain in her knees, has difficulty sleeping, is always sleepy, feels dizzy, is anemic, has a relapse of her arthritis (or migraines, or any chronic problem), complains of hair loss, change of vision, ringing in the ears, or itchy skin. Breastfeeding will be blamed as the cause of marriage problems and when the other children act up. Breastfeeding is to blame when the mortgage rates go up and the economy is faltering. And whenever there is something that does not fit the "picture book" life, the mother will be advised by everyone that it will be better if she stops breastfeeding.

Chapter Eight

Our Breastfeeding Heritage

There's an old saying, "you must know your past to know your future." The same holds true with breastfeeding and African American women. It's important to understand about our breastfeeding past, to get a better understanding of our current state of breastfeeding, which may lead to a greater acceptance of breastfeeding in the future. Let's look at our rich cultural tradition of breastfeeding through the ages.

It's unfortunate that there is such a void of solid evidence about breastfeeding practices during the early part of our history. Breastfeeding research did not become an area of interest until the early part of the 1900s. Even then, it was not necessarily breastfeeding facts or problems that were of concern. It was not that breastfeeding rates were decreasing. The medical community began to take an interest because of an increase in the research and manufacture of breast milk substitutes—what we now call infant formula. There was also a public health interest in infant health, illness, and mortality, as well as a host of other issues facing women and society at large.

During Slavery

Breastfeeding was part of the African culture for thousands of years. To date, there is little evidence of any breast milk substitutes in early African history. Breastfeeding was a normal part of life. Wet nursing was also normal, and an essential part of daily life. Weaning tended to happen anywhere from two to five years in Ancient Egypt to up to six years in some tribal groups in East Africa. Breastfeeding was a tradition that African women sustained consistently through European invasion and the subsequent slave trade. Please note that while this is not meant to be a lesson on slavery, it's vital for us to look at certain areas of this time in history because it sheds light on the breakdown in our breastfeeding tradition.

Europeans began their domination and devastation of the African continent and her people around the 1400s (give or take a few hundred years, depending on which accounts you read). By the time the slave trade began to flourish between Africa, America, and the Caribbean islands, millions upon millions of African families were broken apart. During the Middle Passage, the time and voyage between the African continent and its final slave port in one of the three major destinations, an estimated 6 million Africans died. Conditions were inhumane. Africans from different regions, speaking different languages and living different cultural traditions were packed like cargo in the hull of the ship. For the months-long journey it took to reach the slave ports, they were rarely allowed on the deck, which means they did not receive fresh air or the sunlight that was a part of all African culture. They were fed slop, and the little water they received was polluted, and transmitted infections and disease of the sort the Africans had not been exposed to. They were not allowed to wash or to expel human waste in a sanitary manner. Eating, sleeping, and defecating were all done in the same location. Many died from the contamination and illnesses this type of environment creates. Still others died from suicide. If allowed on deck, many attempted to throw themselves into the ocean. If a suicide attempt failed, the slave was brutally beaten as an example of what would happen if others attempted to kill themselves.

Pregnant women were forced to give birth to their babies in the same place that they expelled bodily waste. Thousands of babies died, and many mothers killed their babies to protect them from such a cruel fate.

Once slaves arrived in America or on one of the Caribbean islands, conditions were far from improved. Families were separated, tribes were scattered, and abuse continued. Women were beaten, fondled, raped, and forced onto public display. Mothers with breastfeeding young were lucky if they were allowed to stay together. During the early years of the slave trade and colonization, the African was almost completely stripped of any power.

On plantations, reproduction rights and all things maternal—care of children, decisions about child rearing—were stripped from the African woman. Her ability and decision to reproduce was under the rule and domain of the slave master. She could not decide when to have children, the number of children she wanted, nor any decision related to infant feeding. She could no longer participate in the selection of a husband, as she may have done in Africa. She was not prepared for mothering and marriage with traditional rituals and female rites of passage. The very part of her that made her a distinct person, her femininity, was not under her control.

Marriage between slaves was illegal without the prior knowledge and consent of the slave master. More often than not, slaves were not allowed to marry. They were, however, forced to mate, breed, and reproduce with whomever the slave master chose. He selected which man and woman would be together. His decision was not based on love or compatibility. It was based on the product of two strong slaves, which would mean offspring that would add to slave labor. By controlling marriage and male-female relationships, not to mention breaking up families and selling children to other plantations, the slave master could control slave behavior. Since families were broken and relationships were selected by him, he could keep slave revolts, escape, and uprising to a minimum. With so much change within the slave community, family was not long-term. It was often brief and fleeting.

Slave women either worked in the slave master's (main) house or in the field. Neither placement was better or worse than the other. Both slaves' lives revolved around the slave master, his wife (mistress of the house), and their children.

The slave woman who worked in the house:

- ❖ lived in the main house and slept under the bed of the mistress or with the children.
- ❖ was on duty twenty-four hours a day.
- ❖ cooked and tended the chickens and dairy production.
- ❖ cleaned the main house.
- ❖ made, mended, and washed clothes.
- ❖ cared for minor medical issues within the main house.
- ❖ was the personal maid of the mistress: she washed and styled the mistress' hair, helped her dress, took care of any of the mistress's personal needs and wants, and delivered her babies.
- ❖ nurtured, disciplined, and played with the mistress's children.
- ❖ breastfed/wet-nursed the mistress's children.

The slave woman who worked in the field:

- ❖ was in the field before the sun came up, and left the field long after the sun set.
- ❖ performed hard labor, including the cultivation of cotton, rice, corn, sugar, silk, and indigo.
- ❖ planted and harvested crops, and farmed animals.
- ❖ managed the slave housing, including cooking, cleaning, washing, making and mending clothes, and caring for and breastfeeding the children.

These tasks were physically and mentally exhausting. On top of the back-breaking, labor-intensive life of the slave woman, she habitually had to not just nurture and take care of the needs of the slave master's children, but she also had to give them life with her breast milk, generally for up to two years.

The close bond that breastfeeding creates between a mother and child, or a woman and a baby, is absolute. It's only natural then, that the slave women and the slave master's children would develop close bonds that lasted into adulthood.

The slave woman couldn't breastfeed her own baby on demand, as is important for the health of any newborn. She only had one day "free" of her slave duties. This was the day that she gave birth. She returned to work the day after! She usually had less than twenty-four hours to spend time bonding with and breastfeeding her baby. She could only nurse her baby, generally, two to three times a day. If she was lucky, she was allowed to carry the baby with her in the fields, which allowed her to nurse while she worked. This only lasted for a short period of time, probably a matter of weeks.

Breastfeeding while working was physically challenging, as she was already on her feet for the entire day. This regulated breastfeeding yielded many, many unhealthy babies whose growth was underdeveloped, yielding a generation of short slaves. The slave woman's diet, workload, and regulated feedings led to high infant mortality in the slave quarters. Most plantations allowed slaves to eat two to three times a day. Slaves lived on a meager and unwholesome diet of rationed cornmeal, pork, and molasses. They rarely received fresh meat, fruit, and vegetables.

Slave women were forced to feed their young regular food much too soon, since their breastfeedings were controlled by the slave master. Infants were given a mixture of cow's milk, corn bread, molasses, and the liquid from cooked greens. We know now that almost 100 percent of the African American population is lactose intolerant, or unable to digest the lactose (sugar) found in cow's milk. The cow's milk used was often toxic and full of pollutants. If milk was not used, then contaminated water (slaves did not have access to natural or clean water) replaced it.

This "food" was devoid of the proper vitamins, minerals, proteins, and antibodies vital for an infant. Again, there was a high rate of infant mortality because of disease and starvation. Slavery was a business, and with any business, you want to increase your product. In this case, human life was the commodity. Slave masters were more concerned about increasing numbers; so, if infants were dying, they just increased the pregnancies of the slave women.

Weaning tended to happen between nine and twelve months. Some weaning occurred within just a few months if the mother's milk was of poor quality. Since breastfeeding is a natural form of birth control when feedings are not interrupted, child spacing can be optimal. However, many slave owners deliberately shortened a slave woman's lactation so that she could get pregnant again and deliver more slave labor. Infants who still needed breast milk were sent to a wet nurse; a slave, of course, whose sole job may have been breastfeeding the slaves' and slave master's children. Thousands of slave women died during or soon after childbirth because of malnutrition and the effects of hard labor on pregnancy. Early weaning was particularly harmful for the slave infant because of the unsanitary, infectious conditions associated with living in slave quarters.

The average age for a slave woman to give birth was in her teens. It was not unusual for a slave woman to give birth to up to fifteen babies or more; yet she may have had a large number of miscarriages. Slave women who delivered many babies were considered "good breeders" and tended to have longevity on a plantation, whereas slave women who could not yield a large number of babies were sold quickly. Once a slave girl reached adolescence and childbearing age, she became of interest for her breeding ability and sexuality. Slave women of all ages were easy prey for slave masters, and birthed generations of biracial slave children.

Imagine, for a moment, the emotional and psychological effect of giving birth to your slave master's children, breastfeeding them, and all the while breastfeeding the children of your mistress and slave master. At this point in our history, breastfeeding had to begin its slow demise in our community. Slavery redefined breastfeeding. For us, breastfeeding was once a traditional, normal part of being a mother—an extension of pregnancy and childbirth. It was a necessity that involved the love and care of our babies, with weaning around age three. Once reaching these shores, breastfeeding began to deviate from being an act of love to the brutality of the slave experience.

Mothering and the slave woman had two dimensions: the external part, based on her condition in slavery; and the internal part, based on her mind and emotions. Superficially, on a very basic level, the slave woman's role as a mother was nonexistent. She was a gateway for her child's birth, and nothing more. This was carefully orchestrated by the slave master to increase his human resources. As mentioned earlier, her sole duty was to do what the slave master required of her, including field work, reproduction, wet-nursing, and sex. She could not choose when to breastfeed, when to start solids, how to care for a sick child, who the child would marry, where he/she could go or who they could play with, what the child would be when he/she grew up. Just as her basic rights as a human were stripped from her, so was her experience with mothering. The usual nurturing that is part of being a mother was not a part of the slave woman's experience. She worked long hours and had little time to spend with her children. She had, at best, brief moments in the morning before work, and brief moments at night after work to focus on mothering. The mother-child bond that is critical for emotional healing for women, and psychological development of children, was almost nonexistent.

Breastfeeding Post-Slavery

After over two-hundred-fifty years of brutality, slavery officially ended in 1863, with most slaves not set free until years later. For many years, although slavery was against the law, it was still practiced. Even after the Civil War ended, and slaves were freed in large numbers, their plight was still dreadful.

A small victory of freedom was the regaining of some control over their lives, particularly in the area of marriage and childbirth. Family was once again a true part of our frame of reference, and familial roots could be planted. Yet, this was short-lived, as racism was still an epidemic that plagued our community. And, with larger societal problems—world wars—the family took another hit. We moved from finally having two parents in the home to one or both parents leaving to find work. Money was difficult to earn, so parents had to go to the North during the Great Migration, or back to sharecropping for months at a time to provide for their families. Black babies were left in the care of older family members. African American babies were forced, once again, to take breast milk substitutes that were nutritionally unsafe and devoid of antibodies—leading to increased Black infant mortality.

Many African American women worked the same types of positions they held during slavery, with the exception of being free. Wet nursing was still a part of her frame of reference in the early part of the 1900s. The pay for this type of position was deplorable. In 1912, the *Independent* newspaper quoted a forty-year-old Black nanny as saying, "Perhaps a million of us are introduced daily to the privacy of a million chambers throughout the South, and hold in our arms a million white children, thousands of whom, as infants, are suckled at our breasts—during my lifetime I myself have served as wet nurse to more than a dozen white children. In the distant future, it may be centuries and centuries hence, a monument of brass or stone will be erected to the Old Black Mammies of the South; but what we need is present help, present sympathy, better wages, better hours, more protection, and a chance to breathe for once while alive as free women. If none others will help us, it would seem that the Southern white women themselves might do so in their own defense, because we are rearing their children—we feed them, we bathe them, we teach them to speak the English language, and in numberless instances we sleep with them—and it is inevitable that the lives of their children will in some measure be pure or impure, according as they are affected by contact with their colored nurses."

She mentioned later in the article that her thirteen-year-old daughter was employed as a wet nurse and paid $1.50 a week. After slavery ended, most women employed as wet nurses were Black or poor women. During this time, the breast milk from wet nurses—who were largely African American—was determined to be inadequate for white babies. Human milk banks accepted breast milk from Black women with reservations, once again, about its quality for white babies. It would appear that to the medical community and affluent white mothers, breast milk was a commodity that was essential for health reasons, and had little to do with bonding and nurturing a baby.

The late nineteenth and early twentieth centuries also brought new advancements in medical technology. There was a shift from home births and midwives to hospital-based deliveries, medications during labor, and infant formula use. Physicians began to discourage the use of wet nurses and midwife services. Up to that time, all births—for Black and white women—happened at home. Black women were assisted either by a sister, mother, friend, or the "woman who caught babies." Today, she'd be called a midwife. Hospital births were generally considered by the public as unsanitary. Women who delivered in hospitals were from low economic groups, who were given free services and chiefly acted as guinea pigs for the medical profession.

By the nineteenth century, the practice of midwifery and home births was in the minority, and hospital births began a road to normalcy. The late nineteenth century brought with it two drugs to ease the pain of childbirth. Many women were routinely put to sleep during childbirth, and those drugs have advanced to widespread use of a variety of pain relievers during childbirth today. The popularity of hospital births inevitably increased fees, which pushed many low-income women out of this practice because services were no longer offered for free. Many Black women—not to mention poor whites—especially those in rural areas, still had births at home. Hospital births brought new practices in infant care, including separation of mother from baby, which can inhibit breastfeeding success.

While advances were being made in the area of hospital birthing practices, artificial breast milk, or infant formula, was being developed. One of the first companies to create a safer cow's milk blend was the Walker-Gordon Milk Laboratory. They created a "formula" to make cow's milk more acceptable to an infant's system. Even as early as the 1890s, the company was distributing its product to mothers. In less than ten years, there were Walker-Gordon Milk laboratories in ten cities across the country. More than twenty types of infant formula were produced during the late 1890s. Dairy pasteurization and safe milk storage was still a problem. Early formula did not have quality measures for safe storage, which led to frequent contamination.

Many of these formulas were powders that had to be mixed with water. Back then, public sanitation and safe water were a major heath concern. Often, formula was mixed with unsafe water, leaving a baby open to disease. Formula wasn't fortified with iron until later. Bottles were not yet safe, and adequate sterilization was frequently a problem. Many people made infant formula at home because commercial formula was only affordable for the wealthy. This homemade formula consisted of a can of condensed milk (Carnation or Pet), water, and corn syrup (Karo). This practice was especially common in the African American community as late as the 1950s.

Physicians and formula manufacturers worked hard in the early- to mid-1900s to create an infant formula that emulated the nutrients found in breast milk. Many scientific experiments attempted to duplicate the composition of breast milk. The components of breast milk are still a mystery to the medical community. A wide variety of formula was manufactured by different scientists trying to get it right. By the 1950s, there was such a demand for infant formula that manufacturers created a prepared, concentrated formula at a reduced cost, so that the product could reach the most people. The correlation between the increased mass production of infant formula, the decline in breastfeeding rates, and increased infant mortality is evident.

Today

Breastfeeding rates and statistics did not begin to be measured until the early 1900s. Even then, the studies largely focused on infant mortality, and not breastfeeding. One such study, however, found that in 1912:

- ❖ 54.8 percent of Black mothers breastfed their babies
- ❖ 57.6 percent of white mothers breastfed their babies
- ❖ 25.5 percent of Black mothers were breastfeeding and supplementing
- ❖ 17.6 percent of white mothers were breastfeeding and supplementing
- ❖ 19.7 percent of Black mothers did not breastfeed

The breastfeeding rates of African American women today are the sum total of our experience with slavery, racism, economics, breakdown of the family, limited access to breastfeeding resources, limited education, and lack of support. In recent history and at present, African American women have some of the lowest breastfeeding rates in the country. Up to the turn of the nineteenth century, our breastfeeding rates were higher than today. A look at our breastfeeding rates over the years (since these rates have been documented) is fascinating because it clearly shows that breastfeeding was once a normal, acceptable, and necessary part of mothering in our community. Infant formula was the exception, not the rule. Today, however, infant formula is the norm and breast milk is the exception.

A 2003 published study by Ross Laboratories found:

❖ 48.3 percent of African American women initiate breastfeeding in the hospital.

❖ Only 20 percent of us are breastfeeding at six months.

❖ 70 percent of white women initiate breastfeeding in the hospital.

❖ 64 percent of Hispanic women initiate breastfeeding in the hospital.

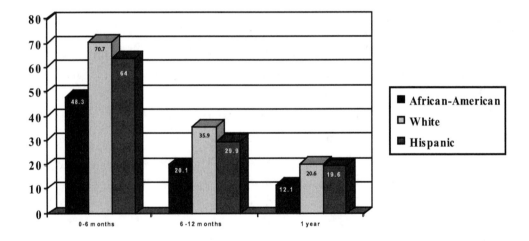

In the new millennium, the African American breastfeeding experience is uncertain. Sadly, our breastfeeding rates today—at a time when information is supposedly accessible to everyone—are nearly the same as in 1923. Only 48 percent of us attempt to breastfeed in the hospital. This rate does not necessarily mean that we are exclusively breastfeeding, but that we attempt to breastfeed. And by six months, barely 20 percent are still breastfeeding. This means that we are giving our babies breast milk in addition to infant formula, whole milk, juice, water, food, and/or other supplements. Even those of us who initiated breastfeeding often did so with the inclusion of infant formula, and not exclusive breastfeeding. We have the lowest initiation and duration of breastfeeding in the country; yet, our babies die more in infancy, and have some of the more acute health problems, including asthma.

There is a general lack of normalcy—something that we see or hear everyday—about breastfeeding in our community. We've seen our breastfeeding history through the ages, and how things like slavery, wet-nursing, and harsh conditions affected our tradition. Now, we have many generations of babies born without the benefit of breast milk. We don't have women in our community whom we can call and ask breastfeeding questions, or whom we can look to as breastfeeding role models. There are a few African American celebrities who have been open about their support of breastfeeding, but they are few. R&B singers Lauryn Hill and Brandy both have voiced their belief in the importance of breastfeeding. Actress Hollie Robinson Peete successfully breastfed twins. Actress and singer Jada Pinkett Smith breastfed both of her children. Magic Johnson and Michael Jordan, sports heroes and businessmen, were both breastfed.

Yet, we still don't have women in our everyday lives—at the beauty or nail salon, doctor's office, mall, library, bus, subway—who breastfeed. We simply don't see it enough. Even when we read breastfeeding literature or watch videos, we don't see images of us, in all our many hues, breastfeeding. We always see white or Hispanic women breastfeeding, in literature and in public. Images of Black women breastfeeding are generally pictures from tribal groups in Africa—women whose breasts are stretched out, and whose bodies are undernourished. These images do little to encourage Black women to breastfeed because we can't relate to the tribal woman.

We have a rapidly growing number of teenage mothers. They are even less likely to breastfeed, often considering breastfeeding as "nasty" or confining. The older and more educated an African American woman is, the more likely she is to breastfeed, and for a longer period of time. There are small pockets of us around the country who have embraced breastfeeding, but the numbers are scattered. We tend to be the only ones in our community who breastfeed. Black stay-at-home moms (see Mocha Moms in the resource section) are more likely to breastfeed as well. Black women who decide to breastfeed tend to be staunch breastfeeding supporters. We are powerful voices in our community for breastfeeding promotion.

The Future

What's ahead for breastfeeding in the African American community? That's up to each one of us. It will take the voice of each Black woman who breastfeeds. You'll need to share your experiences and knowledge with other women. You should support your sisters who become pregnant and who are breastfeeding. It will mean stepping out of your comfort zone and talking about breastfeeding as a very real and essential part of mothering. So often we freely share information about infant formula, clothing, toys, strollers, and car seats. We should share breastfeeding information in the same manner.

If you are reading this book as a father, friend, grandmother, or health care or lactation professional, you can play an important role in the future of breastfeeding in our community. You can support women who choose to breastfeed, and share information with anyone you know who plans to breastfeed. Your promotion of breastfeeding as a doctor, spouse, or friend can make a difference. The more people talk about breastfeeding, the more it becomes normal, as opposed to a strange activity that only a few women experience.

If more African American women would breastfeed, then we would see a remarkable increase in the health of our babies, and decreased infant mortality, asthma, childhood diabetes, etc. Healthy babies often become healthy adults, which means a healthier African American community. Even beyond the health benefits to our babies and ourselves, breastfeeding will increase our self-esteem. Imagine a community of empowered African American women. That will trickle down into our roles in our families, the workplace, and society as a whole. Breastfeeding is a win-win situation for our community.

Chapter Nine

Self-Empowerment through Breastfeeding

In previous chapters, you've read about all the amazing benefits of breast-feeding for you, your baby, and society as a whole. You know that breast milk protects your baby from a long list of diseases; and that breastfeeding protects you from certain types of cancer and other health issues. There's one additional benefit of breastfeeding, however, that receives little attention. Did you know that breastfeeding can help to improve your self-esteem, and give you a sense of self-empowerment? Let's break this idea down, bit by bit, so you can see that breastfeeding goes much deeper than providing nourishment for your baby. Later in the chapter, you'll read stories about women, just like you, who have been empowered through breastfeeding. You'll hear from a mother who successfully breastfed twins; as well as other honest, heartfelt, and encouraging stories from women just like you.

Self-Empowerment

Self-empowerment means having power over your life. Breastfeeding is one of the purest forms of empowerment for women. When you choose to breastfeed, you are demonstrating to the world—or at least your own environment—that you are empowered and have the strength to take on your own destiny. You may or may not be a nuclear engineer or a doctor.

You have power, however, right at your disposal (breast milk) to ensure the most optimal health for your child. Through the "womanly art of breast-feeding," you have the power to offer your child something that no one else can: nutrition, bonding, and immunity to illnesses. Breastfeeding empowers you to believe that Y-O-U can do anything.

Self-Actualization

As Black women, we have a beautiful heritage of resilience, strength, and progress. Breastfeeding helps women begin to fully realize their potential. The decision to breastfeed is not always an easy one to make, because of societal norms that don't include breastfeeding, and because of the monopoly formula companies have on infant food choices—formula and formula-based foods. When you choose to breastfeed, you are, in essence, going against the status quo of many societal, and often familial, customs. By going "outside the box," breastfeeding mothers can begin to understand that the simple act of breastfeeding is only the start of what they can truly achieve in their lives.

Did you ever say as a child, "When I grow up, I want to be a teacher, doctor, dancer, lawyer, or astronaut?" (Or fill in the blank with whatever, you get the meaning here.) Did you ever dream of owning your own business, traveling around the world, or being able to shop for anything you want? Did you have a passion for helping people, saving animals, or making a difference in the world? Did you ever know, deep down inside, that you could do great things during your lifetime? Well, the answer to these questions is quite simply your potential—what you believe you have the ability to do. Self-actualization is a big term with a pretty basic meaning: to realize or know your potential, and to become what you dream you have the ability to accomplish. In short, it means believing something about yourself and making it happen. To help you understand this concept of self-actualization, here are some characteristics of self-actualized people, or people who achieve their potential. These people tend to:

❖ be optimistic and comfortable in their skin, or at least try to be.

❖ accept their own faults.

❖ have self-respect and respect others.

❖ be honest and compassionate.

❖ reach for goals, enjoying success as each part of the journey.

So, how do self-actualization and breastfeeding work together? When you decide to breastfeed, you are setting a goal, which is to provide optimal nutrition and bonding for your baby. You succeed, and actually see your goal accomplished. It does not matter if you breastfeed for a matter of days, weeks, months, or years. You accomplish greatness by breastfeeding your baby, and create a legacy of health and bonding between you and your child that lasts a lifetime. In fact, if you have a daughter, she'll likely breastfeed her own children, and your legacy will continue.

Self-Esteem

Breastfeeding builds self-esteem. As a breastfeeding mother, you will deal with issues from total attachment to your baby to finding discreet ways to nurse in public. You will be forced to acquire a certain level of self-esteem and confidence in your own abilities to manage the pressures that can accompany breastfeeding. It also builds self-esteem because you know, unequivocally, that you are offering your child the absolute best form of nourishment, with benefits that last a lifetime.

Self-esteem is the confidence, respect, and satisfaction you find within yourself. It means loving yourself, just the way you are, including your weaknesses. *You* have to like you. It can only come from inside you. It cannot be based on how your mate, friends, family, boss, coworkers, neighbors, or doctors feel about you. It's the very foundation that sets the stage for happiness or misery. Self-esteem can make or break your life experiences. It plays a role in how you handle the ups and downs of life.

Self-esteem deals with how you feel about your values, your emotions, your innermost feelings, and your physical body. If you have high self-esteem, you'll go far in life, because you have a positive view of yourself and won't let outside forces crush your determination and belief in yourself. High self-esteem will allow you to make it through tough times in life, like experiencing breastfeeding challenges, without being crushed. The characteristics of a person with high self-esteem are:

❖ loving and accepting yourself;

❖ confidence;

❖ forgiveness of yourself and others;

❖ good health; and

❖ an ability to bounce back from challenges.

Low self-esteem often leads to negative life experiences and depression, with a poor quality of life and unhealthy views of oneself, and an inability to see the bright side of any situation. While self-esteem comes from within, it is often shaped and affected by childhood experiences, family, and society. High self-esteem does not mean a perfect life, but it means that you'll be able to cope with the ups and downs, including those that may come with breastfeeding.

Leslie Sherrod's Story
Stay-at-Home Mom, Writer
Husband: Brian Sherrod
Children: Neyla (4, breastfed for fourteen months) and
**   Nathan (2, breastfed for twelve months)**

This was not the scene I studied in the parenting magazines: fully decked out and dimmed nursery, plush rocking chair and ottoman, nursing baby staring with awe into her mother's beaming blue eyes. No, I'm standing in the middle of Harbor Place, a crowded waterside attraction in Baltimore, Maryland, with a six-week-old infant who's crying, and a husband who's pushing around a stroller packed with everything except a bottle, desperately attempting to find a quiet corner for me to calm her down. I was new at this: motherhood, family-of-three outing, breastfeeding.

And what an introduction it had been so far. All the reading and training in the world had not prepared me for the every-two-hours day and night feeding schedule, the explosive engorgements, the prickly-feeling "let-downs," and the occasional three-hour feeding frenzies (yes, I mean three hours of virtual nonstop nursing). What's worse than the fact that I'm trying to learn all this is the fact that my baby girl, Neyla, is learning this also. And she's not looking at me in awe. She's screaming in horror. This was not at all what I imagined when I made the decision to breastfeed. Attracted to the free health benefits of a natural formula—did I say free?—perfected to my child's development, I never realized the work, dedication, and commitment breastfeeding would entail.

But sitting on that bench in the middle of thousands of tourists at Harbor Place, hiding with a blanket the act I would continue for twelve more months, I realized—I knew—I was doing the absolute best thing I could do for my baby. I was doing more than feeding her: I was cuddling her; soothing her in a world brand new to her; establishing a relationship and bond with her that nobody else on this planet could give her. And she knew it.

It was extremely hard, borderline ridiculous, to start the breastfeeding bond those first six weeks. But with the support of my husband, who grew to appreciate the nurture I shared with Neyla, and the support of the women around me who promised this thing would get better to the point of becoming second nature (first nature really), my daughter and I succeeded. It took obstinate determination and patience on my part, gentle prodding and continued learning on Neyla's, but we made it. And now Neyla is a healthy, imaginative three-year-old with an eighteen-month-old brother, Nathan, who also benefited from breast milk for the first year of his life. It was easier the second time around. At six weeks I was nursing that boy without a blink at a dinner party, in a crowded Friday's restaurant, forkful of grilled chicken in one hand, him in the other. I'd also learned to give him Poly-Vi-Sol vitamins to avoid any vitamin D deficiencies, which happened to Neyla (another story, another day, all gone, all good).

To me, the ease that came with ready-made, perfectly heated nutrition was only a bonus to the empowering, relationship-defining, confidence-building, and weight-loss-inducing perks that came with breastfeeding. That time went so quickly, and my life has been forever changed. And yes, those gentle, endearing moments in a dimmed nursery did come. Only I was the one doing the looking into my babies' brown eyes with awe.

Liza Araujo-Rouse's Story

Marketing Analyst
Husband: Patrick Rouse
Children: Gabrielle (8, breastfed for nine months),
**   Sheridan (5, breastfed for six months), and**
**   Logan (1, did not nurse)**

I remember like it was yesterday when I decided to breastfeed. The experience will forever be embossed on my heart. As I anticipated the birth of my first child, I had already made up my mind that I was not going to nurse. I couldn't even fathom the thought of nursing. Believe it or not, in my mind it didn't seem natural, and nothing my girlfriends could say would convince me otherwise. Since my mother's experience with nursing me wasn't a positive one, even her words of encouragement didn't make a difference. I just knew I would feel like a "milked cow."

Sometimes our plans are not what God has in store for us. Gabrielle arrived eight weeks early. After losing two sons prior to having Gabrielle, she was everything we had prayed for and more. Words cannot describe the flood of emotion that poured over me when I first laid eyes on her. However, Gabrielle's early arrival meant an indefinite stay in the National Intensive Care Unit (NICU). The doctor's first prognosis was that she was generally healthy, but still underdeveloped in several areas. He discussed the care she would receive over the next few hours, and asked if I would be breastfeeding. My response was quick and sharp. "Absolutely not!"

He explained that she would benefit greatly if I would simply reconsider. He said I had some time to think about it since they would be feeding her intravenously for the next couple of days. Over the next twelve hours, a lactation specialist tried everything short of harassment to change my mind. On her eighth visit to my bedside, she finally appealed to that instinctual need that most mothers have to protect their young. Her exact words were, "This is the greatest gift you can give to her, and she needs you to get stronger." The next morning a breast pump was sent to my room.

I tried every three hours for two days to express milk from my sore and swollen breasts, but was unsuccessful. Each time I would get maybe five drops of colostrum, and that's being generous. By the third day, I was exhausted, frustrated, and emotionally drained by the entire experience of delivery. In fact, I told the doctors in the NICU to give her formula when they removed the IV and feeding tubes. Once again, the persistence of the lactation specialist won me over. She suggested that we go to visit the baby, and at least try to get her to latch on. The specialist warned me not to get frustrated, because preemies have to *learn* the sucking reflex, and latching on can take time.

Well, to my amazement, Gabrielle latched right on. When she placed her little hand across my heart as she nursed I was reduced to tears. I felt like I was nursing her back to health in the only way I could. We were bonding on a level that cannot be described in words. She needed me, and I was providing. Over the next five months I looked forward to our feeding times together. I felt empowered, and breastfeeding came naturally. It was our quiet time to truly get to know one another, and many times I didn't have to say a word to her. I would gently lay her against my breast and nurture her. Our hearts would sing to one another. I knew instantly that this was the way God meant it to be.

Don't get me wrong, nursing did not come without its challenges, but it was worth the investment. I was investing in my daughter's health and growth. It was that commitment to her well-being that kept me going when I was tired and developed mastitis, a breast infection. I also had the support of my husband and family. Having a strong support system is a must. My family took turns for the first month making meals and cleaning the house to ensure that I was eating properly and getting enough rest; and my husband did everything else. He would get up with me during the midnight feedings just to talk or fetch me a glass of water. Most important, he would encourage me, because he didn't want me to feel like I was on my own in the decision to breastfeed. In addition, the support of the lactation specialist was invaluable! Whenever I had problems or concerns, she was only a phone call away. The experience was made much easier just knowing I had her as a resource. She helped me with everything from positioning to recommending an ointment for cracked nipples to noticing the symptoms of mastitis.

She was also there to discuss my reservations about breastfeeding in public. Nursing in public was probably my biggest challenge. I just wasn't comfortable with the idea. At first, I tried to do everything around the baby's feeding schedule. When I realized that this was next to impossible,

I would either find places that had a women's lounge or nurse in the car. When I had no other choice but to nurse in public, the clothing that supported nursing and the breastfeeding shawl were a godsend. They helped to ease the discomfort.

The decision to nurse had as many advantages as it did challenges. My husband began to see me in whole new light. I wasn't just his wife, but a mother. Strangely, this made him much more endearing. Although the lack of sleep as we adjusted to nursing made getting back to our intimate relationship more difficult, when we did make love, it was more passionate and desirable. I will say that it took some time to really feel comfortable about sharing my body with him and the baby, but my spouse gave me the space I needed. We also talked as much as we could about how we both felt about sex and breastfeeding. This took pulling some teeth, but I was persistent, and he eventually opened up.

Other advantages were the bonding experience with the baby, minimizing the instances of early childhood illnesses, and the fact that we did not have the high cost of formula. The hardest thing about nursing was the weaning process. For me, this experience was not gradual. It was very abrupt, which made it very difficult emotionally and physically. I had planned that when I returned to work, I would express my milk and have the baby-sitter bottle-feed the baby. In the evenings I would nurse her. This was an awesome idea in theory. In reality, it did not work. Once I introduced the bottle, the baby would no longer accept my breast. This happened over a period of about a week. When I tried to nurse her, she would act as if she could not latch on. When I spoke to the specialist, she confirmed that the baby had nipple confusion, a very common condition in preemies. Apparently, it was easier for her to latch on to the bottle than the breast. I was devastated. I cried for weeks. I felt like my heartstrings had been ripped from me. I was terrified that I had disrupted the bonding process and she would suffer from it. Physically, I was in pain. My breasts were engorged and on fire. They ached for days.

However, once my head stopped spinning I realized that, though I had only nursed for a few months, I had given her a wonderful start. Born a preemie, Gabrielle is now a happy, healthy second grader. She is thriving and not as susceptible to illness. I will never regret my decision. In fact, I thank God that he used the lactation specialist as a vessel to speak to me. As a result, when I had my second child, breastfeeding was the only way!

Michelle McIlwaine's Story
Breastfeeding Product Merchant, Lactation Counselor
Husband: Marcus McIlwaine
Children: Marcus Jr. (15, did not nurse)
        Marquise (10, breastfed for one year) and
        twin girls Marquela and Michaela (5, breastfed for nine
        months)

My family was not supportive of breastfeeding in the beginning. I received most of my initial support from my doctor and La Leche League. I didn't breastfeed my first son, but I did with my second. I had not thought about breastfeeding during my pregnancy, so I didn't really have any expectations about the breastfeeding experience. I decided to nurse after he was born. The nurse asked me if I wanted to try it and I said sure.

Once he latched onto my breast, I couldn't imagine any other way to feed him. When Marquise latched on, it felt natural, and there was no pain whatsoever. I was not breastfed, and the only thing my mother ever said to me about breastfeeding was, "It's nasty!" She would say "yuck" every time she saw me nurse my middle son. Later, I found out she added formula to his breast milk on many occasions to thicken it or make him sleep better; her theory, not mine. I was livid, to say the least.

When I gave birth to my twin girls a few years later, I was not confident that I could provide enough breast milk for two babies. I did provide a formula supplement when I felt it was necessary, and at about nine months, they were receiving more formula than breast milk. I worked from home for three weeks postpartum, and then returned to the office when the twins were ten weeks old. Talk about challenging! Keeping up with pumping, caring for two school-aged children along with the twins, being a wife, taking care of our home, and returning to work, whew! Somehow, with prayer, I did overcome the challenge by setting a schedule and getting things prepared the night before.

I was confident about nursing in public. I never really had a problem with that. Usually, though, I only nursed one baby at a time in public. The best part about breastfeeding was looking at the little faces and seeing such love and beauty, and getting a back rub from a tiny little hand. The worst part was the leaking, which several layers of nursing pads helped to control. My husband did eventually support breastfeeding. He didn't like me nursing in public, but if I did he'd have my back and challenge anyone who gave me a second look! As far as our sex life, we had to learn how to work around the leaking breast milk, which was pretty hilarious at times!

With more experience in breastfeeding, I began to talk to other women about it. I let them know it is a sacrifice, but it is one of love, and one of many they will have to make as a mother—but also one of the sweetest. Weaning worked out well, I think, because I often mixed formula and breast milk. My children didn't go cold turkey. I weaned gradually. Breastfeeding changed my life and made me more confident! Knowing that I could provide this gift to my child was priceless.

Having to return to work very early after giving birth made me sad. Nursing required me to spend time with my children, hold them, look into their little faces, and embrace my role as a mother. I just feel like they know me better because of the time we had together during those nursing sessions. The ability to nurture your child by breastfeeding is a divine gift. Receive it!

Dr. Sahira Long's Story
Pediatrician
Husband: Gary Long
Child: Jalen Long (3, breastfed for twelve months)

My husband and immediate family were very supportive. Extended family members were not obviously supportive or against breastfeeding, but lived far enough away that they had little impact in my decision. Prior to ever becoming pregnant, I decided I would attempt to breastfeed any child I gave birth to, after learning the benefits of breastfeeding for mothers and their breastfed babies while working closely with the lactation consultant at GWU Hospital, Nancy Clark, during a nursery rotation in my first year of residency.

I was breastfed. While I was still breastfeeding my son, my mother shared some of her views and experiences during the time she breastfed me after I questioned her. She related that the thing she valued most during the time was the special bond it created between us. I decided to breastfeed because I wanted to give my son the very best I could offer, which, in terms of feeding, meant no formula at all to me. Being a doctor, I knew all the health benefits and felt that breastfeeding would be the least I could do to protect him against all the germs I would bring home from work, and to try to prevent him from inheriting my husband's childhood asthma and allergies. Also, who wouldn't want a smarter child? And emotionally, I wanted to create the bond I'd heard so much about.

I had a few friends that were successful breastfeeding beyond a couple of weeks. I attended one breastfeeding class as a part of a rotation when I wasn't even expecting. My OB never discussed breastfeeding with me, which was one of many other things assumed and never discussed. I had all of the textbook expectations: pain-free as long as I got a good latch; feedings every two to three hours initially; adequate milk supply without offering supplements; successful breastfeeding until the first teeth appeared—when I would be bitten. My first two to three weeks weren't very close to my expectations; I became very good friends with Lansinoh, as my nipples were very sensitive to begin with. The initiation of feeds made me cringe at times, despite my son's seemingly good latch.

In spite of all the breastfeeding assistance I was able to offer parents of newborns at work, I greatly benefited from the encouragement and reassurance offered by a few minutes of hands-on assistance from Nancy Clark (LC extraordinaire) when my sleeping baby refused to wake in the immediate postpartum period. My sleeping angel was transformed into a feeding machine during his first growth spurt, and often attempted to nurse every half hour to an hour, without allowing me time to eat enough to be able to produce the quantity of milk he demanded. Fortunately, with a little help from fenugreek, I was able to maintain my milk supply, even after returning to residency, and only resorted to supplementation when I accidentally left my expressed breast milk at work and had no access to the building after hours. Incidentally, my son's first two teeth erupted at the tender age of four months (with eight by the age of twelve months), and I can't remember a time I was bitten, because I paid careful attention to the end of feedings and promptly ended them when he seemed ready to start playing.

Our first latch took place shortly after Jalen was born in the delivery room, and I either cried or really felt like crying, due to the emotions I experienced. Jalen was extremely alert and opened wide his little mouth, latched with no difficulty, and fed for at least twenty minutes on each side. The love and closeness I felt for him at that moment cannot be described.

For sore nipples, Lansinoh cream is truly a gift from God, as well as altering positions, and doing as little to irritate sore nipples as possible. I was engorged once. My milk came in after three days, at a point when Jalen would sleep for four hours, regardless of our attempts to wake him. I took lots of warm showers, manually expressed and pumped milk, and slept in positions that didn't put pressure on my breasts until they became "smart breasts" and only made the amount of milk he needed. Our sleeping baby turned into a feeding machine with reflux disease. I gave in to demand feedings as long as at least one hour had passed since the last feed and less than four to five hours had passed since the last time I had eaten. I coped with the short downtimes by preparing quick meals that required nothing more than removal from the refrigerator so that I could eat while feeding if needed.

I had to return to work eight weeks after Jalen was born and was scheduled to be on-call the very first day I returned. I had very supportive colleagues who offered a shoulder to cry on if needed, and ample time to pump, but that first night was like torture. I pumped with pictures of Jalen in front of me, and didn't miss an opportunity to show everyone all of the pictures I had taken since he was born. I was confident, but chose to breastfeed discreetly in places where men were present, for my husband's sake. I was refused the use of a dressing room to nurse in at the Gap Outlet in Leesburg, although there were no chairs in the store other than those in the dressing area. I decided that as long as there was a chair, I would nurse whenever and wherever my child was hungry.

The best part about breastfeeding was being able to do something for my child that no one else could do, which made it easier to cope with having to return to work. The worst part was having to pump when I'd much rather be home nursing. I only wore nursing bras, but made sure that my clothes were loose-fitting and two pieces. My husband was very supportive of breastfeeding, simply because it was something I clearly desired to do initially. Once he learned all the benefits of breastfeeding, he became an advocate in our circle of friends, and would offer to talk to friends who were less supportive of their wives' decision to breastfeed. I would occasionally experience a letdown during intimacy that made it difficult to enjoy the act, for fear of inducing another one (I had a very powerful letdown). This, combined with the drying effect breastfeeding had on the vaginal mucus, made for a not-so-pleasant experience. We were able to enjoy sex without a lubricant once I weaned. Fortunately, my OB had already warned that these things might happen, so the latter we were prepared for.

Being a pediatrician, I encourage parents to do what's best for their children, and that includes breastfeeding. I share with them the benefits to each member of the team and provide any assistance I can to help them toward a healthy start. This translates into my private life as well, where I encourage my friends to try to breastfeed, with instructions to call me before they give up. I gradually began weaning when Jalen was close to ten months. The process was made simpler by the fact that I was already working full time, so there were only morning and evening feeds to wean. I would remove one feeding every three weeks or so, until the only one left was his morning feeding that ended on his birthday. I substituted snacks or mealtimes for most of the feedings, and made sure we had just as much cuddle time as we had when he was nursing.

Breastfeeding provided Jalen and me with a bond that I am sure we would not have had if I bottle-fed him. It gave me a way to be close to my child, even when I had to return to work. With personal experience added to the textbook knowledge I had previously, I have become a much more hands-on, vocal advocate of breastfeeding. My experience has given me the desire to become a lactation consultant so I can have knowledge of more tools that can be used to allow more families to successfully breastfeed.

Desiree Eades-Jones's Story
Stay-at-Home Mom
Husband: Calvin Jones
Children: Athenia (8) and Zachary (6), both breastfed eighteen months
My husband and my family supported my decision to breastfeed. My mother-in-law breastfed six of my husband's siblings. I decided to breastfeed when I found out I was pregnant with my oldest, Athenia, although I wasn't a breastfed baby. I decided to breastfeed because it seemed like the natural and reasonable thing to do. My mother told me that she wasn't able to produce milk because of health problems. She says she always regretted not being able to breastfeed. She wonders now with all the new information if she would have been able to breastfeed with the proper help.

For some reason, I wasn't concerned with experiencing breastfeeding problems. Plus, I had lots of help from the NICU staff. I did face a few challenges, though. Pumping for seven weeks while my daughter was in the hospital presented several barriers. Establishing an ample milk supply and sustaining it required lots of diligence. I spent most of my time pumping by hand—even hospital-grade pumps wouldn't work for me. My doctor prescribed Reglan to increase milk production. I wasn't able to wear a bra for the first couple of months because it suppressed my milk production. Even with that challenge, my daughter, who was a preemie, immediately latched on, and it just felt right. Before I became pregnant, I figured I would return to work, but soon found that what I wanted most was to spend time with my baby, which I was fortunate enough to do. Breastfeeding in public never posed a problem for me.

I weaned Athenia during my second pregnancy because nursing became too painful to continue. I would feel some anxiety when I had to leave my daughter, even for a short time, because she refused to eat with anyone else. Honestly, I sometimes felt confined; and early on, I was always stressed about producing enough milk to cover her NICU feedings, which were constantly being increased.

Since my husband was supportive, breastfeeding and our sex life were never at odds for me. There may have been times when I simply wanted my breasts left alone because the baby had been nursing all day. Generally though, it didn't interfere with intimacy. A premature delivery presents lots of challenges with breastfeeding because of the separation from the baby. However, with dedication, they can be overcome, and must, because breast milk is so important to the preterm baby's health and development.

Chapter Ten

Breastfeeding Culture and Politics

At first glance, breastfeeding is simply about feeding and providing the best for your baby. What more could be involved other than latch, position, overcoming barriers, and learning how to breastfeed in public? You might not think that breastfeeding involves more than the bond between you and your baby. Breastfeeding has, in fact, become somewhat of a political issue. As we live in a world governed by politics, no issue is an island in itself. Breastfeeding has global implications, and influences many aspects of daily life.

American Breastfeeding Culture vs. the Rest of the World

The International Labor Organization (ILO) is a United Nations agency that works for social justice and internationally recognized human and labor rights. The ILO formulates international labor standards, setting minimum standards of basic labor rights. In short, it sets principles for companies and employers around the world on how to deal with workers in just and humane ways. More than two-thirds of the world follows the ILO's maternity leave and breastfeeding standards, which suggests:

❖ twelve weeks maternity leave, with extension if necessary.

❖ cash benefits during leave of at least 66 percent of previous earnings.

❖ breastfeeding breaks equal to at least one hour per day.

❖ prevention of dismissal during maternity leave.

Unfortunately, the U.S., a country that many look to for leadership on a variety of issues, does not meet the ILO's standards for maternity leave and breastfeeding. It's now clear that the U.S. has some of the lowest breastfeeding rates of industrialized countries.

Today, the state of the American family is irregular, at best. Where the family was once a societal stabilizer, it is far from what it should be now. Here is data on the U.S. family as of 2000:

❖ 75.3 percent of white children live with married parents

❖ 65.1 percent of Hispanic children live with married parents

❖ 37.6 percent of Black children live with married parents

With many families being led by single parents, especially in the African American community, women often don't get the support they need for successful breastfeeding.

State Breastfeeding Legislation

The battle for breastfeeding legislation has been just that, a battle. Here is some information that may shock you. (Reprinted with permission from *50 States Summary of Breastfeeding Laws* Copyright © 2004 by National Conference of State Legislatures.)

❖ **Only thirty states allow mothers to breastfeed in any public or private location, while the rest have restrictions.** These states are: California, Colorado, Connecticut, Delaware, Florida, Georgia, Hawaii, Indiana, Iowa, Illinois, Louisiana, Maine, Maryland, Minnesota, Missouri, Montana, Nevada, New Hampshire, New Jersey, New Mexico, New York, North Carolina, Oklahoma, Oregon, Rhode Island, South Dakota, Texas, Utah, Vermont, and Virginia.

❖ **Only fifteen states exempt breastfeeding from public indecency laws:** Alaska, Florida, Illinois, Michigan, Montana, Nevada, New

Hampshire, North Carolina, Oklahoma, Rhode Island, South Dakota, Utah, Virginia, Washington, and Wisconsin.

❖ **Ten states have laws related to breastfeeding in the workplace:** California, Connecticut, Georgia, Hawaii, Illinois, Minnesota, Rhode Island, Tennessee, Texas, and Washington.

❖ **Eight states exempt breastfeeding mothers from jury duty:** California, Idaho, Iowa, Minnesota, Nebraska, Oklahoma, Oregon, and Virginia.

❖ **Four states have implemented or encouraged the development of a breastfeeding awareness education campaign:** California, Illinois, Missouri, and Vermont.

Several states have unique laws related to breastfeeding. For instance, California and Texas have laws related to the procurement, processing, distribution, or use of human milk. Louisiana prohibits any child care facility from discriminating against breastfed babies. Maine requires courts, when awarding parental rights and responsibilities with respect to a child, to consider whether the child is under the age of one and being breastfed. Maryland exempts from the sales and use tax the sale of tangible personal property that is manufactured for the purpose of initiating, supporting, or sustaining breastfeeding. Rhode Island requires the Department of Health to prepare a consumer mercury alert notice, explaining the danger of eating mercury-contaminated fish to women who are pregnant or breastfeeding their children.

Behind the Scenes of Breastfeeding Support

Thousands of people across the country and abroad work daily to promote the importance of breastfeeding, support your breastfeeding experience, and protect your right to breastfeed. These individuals, organizations, and government agencies work diligently so that employers can understand the importance of supporting their breastfeeding staff: insurance companies can recognize the need to supplement expenses related to breastfeeding; government agencies can make provisions for breastfeeding in their health agendas; training can be provided for women to help other women with breastfeeding challenges; the public can be made aware of the benefits of breastfeeding; and many, many other important components of keeping breastfeeding as a viable and preferred option for all mothers.

African American Breastfeeding Alliance (AABA)

I founded the African American Breastfeeding Alliance, Inc. (AABA) in 2000 because a disproportionate number of African American women don't breastfeed. For the ones that do try, just about 20 percent breastfeed past six months postpartum. The worldwide average for weaning a child from the breast is four and a half years of age. AABA's mission is to:

❖ increase the number of African American women (and women of African descent) who breastfeed.

❖ educate the African American community about the infant and maternal benefits of breastfeeding.

❖ provide valuable resources about breastfeeding.

❖ offer ongoing support to women who decide to breastfeed.

❖ collaborate with other organizations that have an interest in the health and well-being of African American women and infants.

AABA uses a holistic approach to educating women because breastfeeding is both a mental and a physical experience.

AABA is the first nonprofit organization whose sole purpose is to educate African American women and families about the maternal, infant, and societal benefits of breastfeeding. While there are several websites and books on breastfeeding, none speak directly to the needs of African American women. Goals set by organizations such as the Women, Infants, and Children (WIC) Program and initiatives such as Healthy People 2010 that address the health issues of pregnant and lactating African American women have not created effective interventions to reach these goals. AABA's objectives directly meet the breastfeeding goals of Healthy People 2010. In fact, Healthy People 2010 states on its website that "…increasing the rate of breastfeeding, particularly among the low-income, racial, and ethnic populations less likely to begin breastfeeding in the hospital or to sustain it throughout the infant's first year, is an important public health goal." AABA works to fill the gaps of organizations that have maternal and infant health—specifically breastfeeding—objectives targeting African American women.

AABA targets pregnant women, initially during their second trimester, and then follows up right after the birth with continued breastfeeding support and resources. It has been shown that prenatal clinics offering workshops and information on breastfeeding have a positive influence on African American women who decide to breastfeed. One study suggests, "The prenatal period may be a critical time to influence a prospective black mother's decision to breastfeed her infant." (*JSPN* Vol.1, No. 1, April–June, 1996.) This study also found that "personalized and well-designed educational resources such as pamphlets, brochures, and videos that deal with the benefits, contraindications, and support programs for breastfeeding" prove to be influential in this decision as well.

The dire need for AABA has never been fully explored before. By partnering with health professionals and agencies, AABA is committed to providing quality breastfeeding education, resources, and support to African American women and the health care community at large. Over the past five years, AABA has partnered with the following agencies, organizations, and companies to try to meet the breastfeeding needs of

Black women: the United States Department of Health and Human Services Office on Women's Health, Lansinoh Corporation, La Leche League International, Los Angeles WIC Program, Seattle WIC Program, Morgan State University, and a host of other organizations and agencies. AABA has chapters in Georgia, California, Texas, Washington, DC, and Washington State.

AABA's Projects

The Internet address of AABA is aabaonline.com. The website focuses on the following areas:

- ❖ infant, maternal, and societal benefits of breastfeeding
- ❖ how to breastfeed, express, and store breast milk
- ❖ discreet ways to breastfeed in public
- ❖ nutrition and mother's milk
- ❖ latest in breastfeeding research
- ❖ breastfeeding the older baby
- ❖ breastfeeding on the job
- ❖ breastfeeding and the sick child
- ❖ personal narratives from breastfeeding mothers
- ❖ support and encouragement
- ❖ questions answered
- ❖ resources for further education

The website is not only for the African American breastfeeding mother. It will also be a site where lactation professionals can order culturally sensitive brochures, posters, and publications related to lactating African American women.

An Easy Guide to Breastfeeding for African American Women, a booklet on the basics of breastfeeding, has been distributed across the country. It is available free of charge, and can be found online at aabaonline.com. Also available free of charge is *The Love of Breastfeeding Your Baby*, a collaboration between AABA and Lansinoh. Brochures and newsletters for lactation professionals and breastfeeding women are also available.

The Breastfeeding Drop-In Clinic (BDC) is offered onsite at various agencies and hospitals that do not currently offer lactation services, but want to promote breastfeeding. Currently, there is one in Washington, DC. The BDC provides the following services:

❖ basic breastfeeding management (offered bedside or upon discharge if located in a hospital)

❖ brochures and other materials (for additional breastfeeding management)

❖ breastfeeding hotline (to answer questions and offer support)

❖ breastfeeding aids (pump rentals, supplemental nursing systems, etc.)

❖ postnatal follow-up phone call (to check on how well breastfeeding is going)

❖ basics of breastfeeding in-service training (for labor and delivery staff)

❖ formal assessment and report on each patient seen for the agency's records

In addition, we offer the following support groups and opportunities:

❖ **Mother/Sister Support Groups.** When a woman decides to breastfeed, support is vital to a successful experience. The support groups meet monthly to offer loving support and information to breastfeeding African American women. The meetings are designed to last two hours, during the evening or on the weekends, to accommodate the working mother's schedule.

❖ **Peer Counselor Training.** It has been found that peer counselors are effective in helping African American women continue to breastfeed after initiation. AABA trains women to be peer counselors. This four-day training includes sessions on: anatomy of the breast, composition of breast milk, breastfeeding management, benefits, overcoming barriers, and a host of other issues. The peer counselors are then given opportunities to help women in their own communities.

❖ **Breastfeeding Information Center.** This hotline offers support and counseling to breastfeeding mothers from nine in the morning until five in the evening, Monday through Friday. Call toll-free, (877) 532-8535.

❖ **Lactation Career Path.** We encourage African American women to pursue training and certification as peer counselors, certified lactation educators, and international board-certified lactation consultants. We provide mentors to women who choose to pursue a career in lactation.

Baby-Friendly Hospital Initiative (BFHI)

A baby-friendly hospital means much more than providing quality care to babies and their families. The Baby-Friendly Hospital Initiative (BFHI) is an international program whose mission is to encourage and recognize hospitals and birthing centers that offer an optimal level of care for breastfeeding. BFHI helps hospitals and birthing centers give breastfeeding mothers the information and skills they need to successfully breastfeed. BFHI also gives special recognition to hospitals and birthing centers that have offered a superior level of breastfeeding support. BFHI promotes, protects, and supports breastfeeding through the "Ten Steps to Successful Breastfeeding for Hospitals," designed by WHO/UNICEF:

1. Maintain a written breastfeeding policy that is routinely communicated to all health care staff.

2. Train all health care staff in skills necessary to implement this policy.

3. Inform all pregnant women about the benefits and management of breastfeeding.

4. Help mothers initiate breastfeeding within one hour of birth.

5. Show mothers how to breastfeed and how to maintain lactation, even if they are separated from their infants.

6. Give infants no food or drink other than breast milk, unless medically indicated.

7. Practice "rooming in"—allow mothers and infants to remain together twenty-four hours a day.

8. Encourage unrestricted breastfeeding.

9. Give no pacifiers or artificial nipples to breastfeeding infants.

10. Foster the establishment of breastfeeding support groups, and refer mothers to them on discharge from the hospital or clinic.

The Baby-Friendly USA, which began in 1997, is a nonprofit organization that implements the BFHI, and is sponsored by WHO/UNICEF. Currently, there are forty-two baby-friendly hospitals, and they are in the following states: California, Connecticut, Florida, Hawaii, Idaho, Indiana, Kentucky, Maine, Montana, Nebraska, New Hampshire, New York, Ohio, Oregon, Pennsylvania, Rhode Island, Tennessee, Vermont, Washington, and Wisconsin.

So, why should a birthing facility become baby-friendly? Ultimately, the hospital will be one that provides for the best foundation, optimal start, and lifelong health of infants through the support and promotion of breastfeeding. There are also many benefits to receiving recognition as baby-friendly:

❖ **Quality improvement.** Many of the ten steps are easily adaptable as QI projects.

❖ **Cost containment.** Increased breastfeeding rates can have an impact on many health care costs, from postpartum hemorrhage to decreased incidence of infant ear infection.

❖ **Public relations/marketing.** Families who feel adequately supported during the vulnerable postpartum days can speak powerfully for a birth facility.

❖ **Prestige.** The receipt of this international award is an achievement to celebrate.

To find out more about BFHI, or to apply, visit www.babyfriendly.com or call (508) 888-8092.

La Leche League International (LLLI)

What happens when you connect mothers with a vision and a mission to support each other in breastfeeding and promote its importance to other mothers? La Leche League International (LLLI) is the outcome of a small group of empowered women. A group of women met on October 17, 1957, in Illinois, to talk about the state of breastfeeding. Within two years, they had incorporated and published the first in a long line of publications, *The Womanly Art of Breastfeeding*. Within seven years, their meetings grew to over fifty women, and they instituted their chapter format. LLL then went international, with chapters in four other countries. LLL has established itself as a primary source of breastfeeding information for women and professionals, with a large list of publications and teaching modules. When you think of breastfeeding support around the world, LLL instantly comes to mind. With support groups, many women find breastfeeding support and help from LLL leaders. For more information on LLL, call (847) 519-7730, or visit www.lalecheleague.org.

World Health Organization/United Nations Children's Fund (WHO/UNICEF)

The World Health Organization (WHO) is the United Nations' specialized agency for health. It was established on April 7, 1948. WHO's objective, as set out in its constitution, is the attainment by all peoples of the highest possible level of health. Health is defined in WHO's constitution as a state of complete physical, mental, and social well-being, and not merely the absence of disease or infirmity. UNICEF is the driving force that helps build a world where the rights of every child are realized. This makes UNICEF unique among world organizations, and unique among those working with the young. They believe that nurturing and caring for children are the cornerstones of human progress. UNICEF was created to work with others to overcome the obstacles that poverty, violence, disease, and discrimination place in a child's path. WHO/UNICEF's strategy for infant and toddler feeding is based upon the Innocenti Declaration for the protection, promotion, and support of breastfeeding. The Innocenti Declaration was adopted in 1990. The aim is to create an environment, globally, that empowers women to breastfeed exclusively for the first six months, and continue to breastfeed for two years or more. This is optimal infant and toddler feeding, the best start to life. It is expected to improve the nutrition status, growth and development, health, and thus the survival of infants and young children. It is closely linked to the related maternal nutrition that safeguards women's own well-being.

Perhaps the first international, unified policies to protect breastfeeding began with the World Health Assembly (WHA). In 1981, WHA produced the International Code of Marketing of Breast Milk Substitutes (The Code), which sets a guideline for interested individuals and organizations to respond to the marketing of infant formula (or any breast milk substitute) and infant bottles, or teats.

The Code states that:

❖ There should be absolutely no promotion of breast milk substitutes, bottles, or teats to the general public.

❖ Neither health facilities nor health professionals should ever have a role in promoting breast milk substitutes.

❖ Free samples should not be provided to pregnant women, new mothers, or their families.

The Code is intended for the purpose of regulations to monitor the marketing of infant formula. Government agencies around the world are encouraged to use these standards of practice to further ensure the protection of breastfeeding. Below are examples of some implementations of The Code in different countries:

❖ New Guinea—The sale of feeding bottles and other such items is strictly controlled, and there is a ban on advertising these products and infant formula.

❖ Iran—Formula is only available by prescription. Infant formula products use a generic label with no brand names, pictures, or promotional messages.

❖ India—Cans of infant formula are required, by legislation, to use an obvious, highlighted warning about the potential harm caused by artificial feeding.

United States Breastfeeding Committee (USBC)

The United States Breastfeeding Committee (USBC) is an organization of organizations. Members represent agencies, nonprofit organizations, and government offices. They meet twice a year to work on projects that protect, promote, and support breastfeeding in the U.S. The USBC published

Breastfeeding in the United States: A National Agenda in 2001. The vision/ mission states, "In order to achieve optimal health, enhance child develop- ment, promote knowledgeable and effective parenting, support women in breastfeeding, and make optimal use of resources, we envision breastfeeding as the norm for infant and child feeding throughout the U.S." This publi- cation outlines a strategic plan with four main goals:

❖ Assure access to comprehensive, current, and culturally appropriate lactation care and services for all women, children, and families.

❖ Ensure that breastfeeding is recognized as the normal and preferred method of feeding infants and young children.

❖ Ensure that all federal, state, and local laws relating to child welfare and family law recognize and support the importance and practice of breastfeeding.

❖ Increase protection, promotion, and support for breastfeeding mothers in the workforce.

U.S. Department of Health and Human Services (DHHS)

The United States Department of Health and Human Services (DHHS) has a history of major initiatives to support breastfeeding. From a national video teleconference on breastfeeding by DHHS to former Surgeon General Dr. C. Everett Koop's report of the *Surgeon General's Workshop on Breastfeeding and Human Lactation* in 1984 to Former Surgeon General Dr. David Satcher's *HHS Blueprint for Action on Breastfeeding* to the current, three-year-long DHHS Office on Women's Health National Breastfeeding Awareness Campaign, the U.S. government has showed an increasing commitment to promoting and supporting the importance of breastfeeding in this country.

The Innocenti Declaration states that breastfeeding is a unique process that:

❖ Provides ideal nutrition for infants and contributes to their healthy growth and development.

❖ Reduces incidence and severity of infectious diseases, thereby lowering infant mortality.

❖ Contributes to women's health by reducing the risk of breast and ovarian cancer, and by increasing the time between pregnancies.

❖ Provides social and economic benefits to the family and the nation.

❖ Provides most women with a sense of satisfaction when successfully carried out.

These benefits increase with increased exclusiveness of breastfeeding during the first six months of life, and thereafter with increased duration of breastfeeding with complementary foods; and program intervention can result in positive changes in breastfeeding behavior.

Therefore, we declare that, as a global goal for optimal maternal and child health and nutrition, all women should be enabled to practice exclusive breastfeeding, and all infants should be fed exclusively on breast milk from birth to four to six months of age. Thereafter, children should continue to be breastfed, while receiving appropriate and adequate complementary foods, for up to two years of age or beyond. This child-feeding ideal is to be achieved by creating an appropriate environment of awareness and support, so that women can breastfeed in this manner.

Attainment of this goal requires, in many countries, the reinforcement of a "breastfeeding culture," and its vigorous defense against incursions of a "bottle-feeding culture." This requires commitment and advocacy for social mobilization, utilizing fully the prestige and authority of acknowledged leaders of society in all walks of life. Efforts should be made to increase women's confidence in their ability to breastfeed. Such empowerment involves the removal of constraints and influences that manipulate perceptions and behavior toward breastfeeding, often by subtle and indirect means. This requires sensitivity, continued vigilance, and a responsive and comprehensive communications strategy involving all media, and addressed to all levels of society.

Furthermore, obstacles to breastfeeding within the health system, the workplace, and the community must be eliminated. Measures should be taken to ensure that women are adequately nourished for their optimal health and that of their families. Furthermore, ensuring that all women also have access to family planning information and services allows them to sustain breastfeeding, and avoid shortened birth intervals that may compromise their health and nutritional status, and that of their children.

All governments should develop national breastfeeding policies and set appropriate national targets for the 1990s. They should establish a national system for monitoring the attainment of their targets, and they should develop indicators such as the prevalence of exclusively breastfed infants at discharge from maternity services, and the prevalence of exclusively breast-fed infants at four months of age. National authorities are further urged to integrate their breastfeeding policies into their overall health and development policies. In so doing they should reinforce all actions that protect, promote, and support breastfeeding within complementary programs, such as prenatal and perinatal care, nutrition, family planning services, and prevention and treatment of common maternal and childhood diseases. All health care staff should be trained in the skills necessary to implement these breastfeeding policies.

By the year 1995, all governments should have: appointed a national breastfeeding coordinator of appropriate authority, and established a multisectoral national breastfeeding committee composed of representatives from relevant government departments, nongovernmental organizations, and health professional associations. Ensured that every facility providing maternity services fully practices all ten of the "Ten Steps to Successful Breastfeeding," set out in the joint WHO/UNICEF statement "Protecting, Promoting, and Supporting Breastfeeding: The Special Role of Maternity Services." Taken action to give effect to the principles and aim of all Articles of the International Code of Marketing of Breast Milk Substitutes and subsequent relevant World Health Assembly resolutions in their entirety; and enacted imaginative legislation protecting the breastfeeding rights of working women, and established means for its enforcement. We also call upon international organizations to:

❖ Draw up action strategies for protecting, promoting, and supporting breastfeeding, including global monitoring and evaluation of their strategies.

❖ Support national situation analyses and surveys, and the development of national goals and targets for action.

❖ Encourage and support national authorities in planning, implementing, monitoring, and evaluating their breastfeeding policies.

Surgeon General's Workshop on Breastfeeding and Human Lactation (1984)

The workshop was organized for breastfeeding professionals and the medical community to come up with a strategy to address the importance of breastfeeding on a national level, and to aid in reaching one of the health objectives of DHHS. The objective stated: "The proportion of women who breastfeed their babies at hospital discharge should be increased to 75 percent, and the percentage of those still breastfeeding at six months of age should be increased to 35 percent." Former Surgeon General, Dr. C. Everett Koop, was a key supporter of the importance of breastfeeding as a health issue. Dr. Koop, who gave the keynote address, charged participants from public, private, and governmental agencies, with the following tasks:

❖ to review progress of past efforts, in both public and private sectors.

❖ to promote breastfeeding.

❖ to assess the state of the art related to factors that enhance and those that inhibit breastfeeding and human lactation.

❖ to determine remaining challenges.

❖ to develop strategies and recommendations in order to facilitate progress toward achieving the 1990 objective.

Six workgroups were formed that recommended the following strategies for reaching the 1990 objectives mentioned above:

❖ **World of Work.** A national breastfeeding promotion initiative directed to all those who influence the breastfeeding decisions and opportunities of women involved in school, job training, professional education, and employment is needed.

❖ **Public Education.** Public education and promotional efforts should be undertaken through the education system and the media. Such efforts should recognize the diversity of the audience, target various economic, cultural, and ethnic groups, and be coordinated with professional education.

❖ **Professional Education.** It is imperative for all health care professionals to receive adequate didactic and clinical training in lactation and breastfeeding, and to develop skills in patient education and the management of breastfeeding.

❖ **Health Care System.** The health care system needs to be better informed and more clearly supportive of lactation and breastfeeding.

❖ **Support Services.** The successful initiation and continuation of breastfeeding will require a broad spectrum of support services involving families, peers, care providers, employers, and community agencies and organizations.

❖ **Research.** An intensified research effort, including a broad range of research studies, is needed to provide data on the benefits and contraindications of breastfeeding among women in the United States. Research is also needed to evaluate strategies/interventions, and to determine progress in achieving goals related to the promotion of breastfeeding.

USBC MEMBER ORGANIZATIONS INCLUDE:
- ❖ Academy for Educational Development
- ❖ Academy of Breastfeeding Medicine
- ❖ African American Breastfeeding Alliance
- ❖ American Academy of Family Physicians
- ❖ American Academy of Nursing
- ❖ American Academy of Pediatrics
- ❖ American College of Nurse-Midwives
- ❖ American College of Obstetricians and Gynecologists
- ❖ American College of Osteopathic Pediatricians
- ❖ American College of Preventive Medicine
- ❖ American Public Health Association
- ❖ Association of Military Surgeons of the United States
- ❖ Association of State & Territorial Public Health Nutrition Directors
- ❖ Association of Women's Health, Obstetric, and Neonatal Nurses
- ❖ Baby-Friendly USA
- ❖ Best Start Social Marketing Inc.
- ❖ Center on Budget and Policy Priorities
- ❖ Coalition for Improving Maternity Services

- DHHS/Centers for Disease Control and Prevention
- DHHS/Food and Drug Administration/Center for Food Safety and Applied Nutrition
- DHHS/Health Resources and Services Administration, Maternal and Child Health Bureau
- DHHS/Office on Women's Health
- Healthy Children 2000 Project
- Human Milk Banking Association of North America
- International Board of Lactation Consultant Examiners
- International Lactation Consultant Association
- La Leche League International
- Lamaze International
- Morgan State University
- National Alliance for Breastfeeding Advocacy—Research, Education, and Legal
- National Association of Pediatric Nurse Practitioners
- National Association WIC Directors
- National Commission on Donor Milk Banking
- National Healthy Mothers, Healthy Babies Coalition
- USDA/Food and Nutrition Services/WIC
- University of California, Los Angeles, School of Public Health
- University of Rochester School of Medicine and Dentistry
- University of Southern California, Keck School of Medicine
- Wellstart International
- Women's International Public Health Network

DHHS Blueprint for Action on Breastfeeding (Blueprint) (2000)

More than fifteen years later, the results of goals set forth during the 1984 Workshop—along with other initiatives—began to take real shape. The health objective for 1990, to increase breastfeeding initiation to 75 percent, had not been reached. In the 1990s, DHHS worked diligently to make early recommendations in the 1980s become more of a viable reality. DHHS contributed to the formation of Healthy Mothers, Healthy Babies and the USBC. It also cosponsored the National Breastfeeding Policy Conference in 1998. The Blueprint emerged from DHHS's history of supporting and creating breastfeeding programs, including the various DHHS reports, the 1990 signing of the Innocenti Declaration on the Protection, Promotion, and Support of Breastfeeding by WHO/UNICEF, and the diligent efforts of breastfeeding supporters across the U.S.

The Blueprint is "an action plan for breastfeeding based on education, training, awareness, support, and research. The plan includes key recommendations that were refined by the members and reviews of the Subcommittee on Breastfeeding during their deliberations of science-based findings. Recognizing that breastfeeding rates are influenced by various factors, these recommendations suggest an approach in which all interested stakeholders come together to forge partnerships to promote breastfeeding…with a significant challenge to reach African American women with culturally appropriate approaches to promote breastfeeding." It is designed to offer effective strategies to private, nonprofit, and government agencies/organizations, as well as individuals in the community, for breastfeeding support and promotion. The Blueprint supports the American Academy of Pediatrics' goal that infants should be fed only breast milk for the first four to six months of life. The Blueprint proposes the following measures be taken by any interested individual or organization.

Health Care System

Train health care professionals who provide maternal and child care on the basics of lactation, breastfeeding counseling, and lactation management during internship residency, in-service training, and continuing education. Assure that breastfeeding mothers have access to comprehensive, up-to-date, and culturally tailored lactation services provided by trained physicians, nurses, nutritionists, and lactation consultants. Establish hospital and maternity center practices that promote breastfeeding, such as the "Ten Steps to Successful Breastfeeding." Develop breastfeeding education for women, their partners and other significant family members during the prenatal and postnatal visits.

Workplace

Facilitate breastfeeding or breast milk expression in the workplace by providing private rooms, milk storage arrangements, adequate breaks during the day, flexible work schedules, and onsite child care facilities. Establish family and community programs that enable breastfeeding continuation when women return to work in all possible settings. Encourage child care facilities to provide quality breastfeeding support.

Family and Community

Develop social support and information resources for breastfeeding women such as hotlines, peer counseling, mother-to-mother support groups, etc. Launch a public-health marketing campaign portraying breastfeeding as normal, desirable, and achievable. Encourage the media to portray breast-feeding as normal, desirable, and achievable for women of all cultures and socioeconomic levels. Encourage fathers and other family members to be actively involved throughout the breastfeeding experience.

The Blueprint is an important document about breastfeeding, where our nation stands on the subject, and recommendations to improve breastfeeding rates. One of the major challenges discussed in the Blueprint is that of the low breastfeeding rates of African American women. It states that, "Increasing the rates of breastfeeding is a compelling public health goal, particularly among the racial and ethnic groups who are less likely to initiate and sustain breastfeeding throughout the infant's first year."

If you combine the strategies outlined in the Blueprint and the work of mothers, individuals, and organizations across the country, you get a growing need for something large-scale to be done about breastfeeding. The summer of 2004 marked a milestone in the promotion of breastfeeding. The DHHS Office on Women's Health (OWH) launched their first ever National Breastfeeding Awareness Campaign aimed at increasing breastfeeding rates of first-time mothers. To highlight the importance of breastfeeding and to encourage more mothers to breastfeed exclusively for six months, DHHS/OWH and the AD Council (a nonprofit organization that produces PSAs and is famous for campaigns such as "Only You Can Fight Forest Fires," and "Friends Don't Let Friends Drive Drunk," among others) teamed up to develop this forty-million-dollar breastfeeding awareness campaign.

The campaign is also DHHS's answer to recommendations in the Blueprint. The overall goal of the campaign is to increase the proportion of mothers who breastfeed their babies in the early postpartum period to 75 percent, and those within six months postpartum to 50 percent by the year 2010. This comprehensive three-year media campaign is the first of this magnitude in the breastfeeding community. It includes public service announcements (PSA) for TV, radio, cable, Internet, bus stop shelters, newspapers, magazines, and billboards. The campaign slogan is "Babies Were Born to Be Breastfed." The PSA is distributed across the country and in Puerto Rico.

To provide support for women who view these ads, OWH funded eighteen community-based demonstration projects (CDPs) throughout the U.S. to implement the campaign at the local level. The CDPs include breastfeeding coalitions, hospitals, universities, state health departments, and other organizations. They have been funded to: increase their existing breastfeeding services; provide outreach to their communities; train health care providers on breastfeeding; implement the media aspects of the campaign; and track breastfeeding rates in their communities. The CDP cities are: Atlanta, Birmingham, Boston, Camden, Chicago, Kansas City, Knoxville, Los Angeles, New Orleans, Philadelphia, Portland, Providence, Pueblo, Rosebud, San Francisco, San Juan, St. Paul, and Washington, DC.

Breastfeeding advocates began getting excited as the news of the campaign and its goals began to unfold. A campaign of this nature was sure to be the impetus to make a dramatic shift in breastfeeding rates and support, many assumed. However, a major change occurred. What could be less controversial than breastfeeding? Originally, the goal of the campaign was to focus on the risks of not breastfeeding. These risks include: higher chance of diabetes, obesity, leukemia, recurrent ear infections, diarrhea, asthma, pneumonia, and other respiratory diseases.

Infant formula companies, however, got wind of the campaign before it even started, and put pressure on the government to change it. The campaign was slated to start in early winter, 2003. Another ad showed pregnant women skating at a roller derby. The slogan read, "You wouldn't risk your baby's health before it's born. Why start after?" The implication being that your baby's health is at risk if you don't breastfeed. Other ads duplicated this same sentiment. Infant formula companies saw the ads before they were officially released, and responded with all the force that their two-billion-dollar-a-year industry could muster.

Ultimately, the tone of the ads changed. It went from the risks of not breastfeeding to the benefits of breastfeeding, which is the same approach breastfeeding advocates have taken for the past twenty years. The risk-based approach was necessary because telling women "breast is best" has not been the most effective approach to increasing breastfeeding rates. A stronger, more bold approach is vital for the message to be received. Formula representatives met privately with DHHS Secretary Tommy Thomson and aired their concerns, which they say is not about the importance of breastfeeding —which they supposedly support—but about the implication of a risk-based approach. They claimed that the science behind the campaign was invalid.

One such supporter said, "Many mothers simply cannot breastfeed, or cannot do so for as long as would be desired, or elect not to do so for persuasive reasons (often economic). For our government to give all those mothers a guilt-trip would just be appalling," stated lobbyist Clayton Yeutter, who was hired by the infant formula industry to address this campaign. Dr. Jay Gordon, a pediatrician in Santa Monica, California, and a member of the breastfeeding committee of the American Academy of Pediatrics says, "When you say, 'not breastfeeding is risky,' what you're saying is, 'using infant formula is risky,' and that is true, and they know it." Suddenly, a campaign that was on the verge of starting was halted, and did not launch until six months later, with what many breastfeeding advocates feel was a much watered-down approach. They believe that the current campaign is evidence of the power infant formula companies have in the government and economy. Secretary Thompson did not meet with breastfeeding advocates until long after he met with formula reps and agreed to change the tone of the campaign. The official word out of Secretary Thompson's office, however, was that the campaign was changed because the research was inaccurate. This is pretty hard to believe since the campaign was at least three years in the making with the best medical researchers and breastfeeding experts providing professional consultation on the data used to reach conclusions about breastfeeding.

To the campaign's credit, however, it is still the only effort of such magnitude with the goal of increasing breastfeeding rates. The effect of this campaign can only bring positive attention to breastfeeding. The campaign was ultimately successful at getting people openly talking about breastfeeding—especially those in communities that normally would not breastfeed: ours. Hopefully, pregnant women will see the PSAs and at least consider breastfeeding, and perhaps take the information to their health-care provider for further discussion and education. Even looking at the turn the campaign made in its focus, that attention still helped get people talking about breastfeeding. The result of the campaign will take time to measure. Those out there supporting breastfeeding women, regardless how the campaign works out, are the real heroes. The Office on Women's Health should be applauded for their efforts and continued hard work to promote breastfeeding and fund support when many other agencies won't.

Women, Infants, and Children's Program (WIC)

The WIC target population are low-income, nutritionally at-risk pregnant women, through pregnancy and up to six weeks after birth or after pregnancy ends; breastfeeding women (up to infant's first birthday); non-breastfeeding, postpartum women (up to six months after the birth of an infant or after pregnancy ends); infants (up to first birthday); and children up to their fifth birthday. WIC serves 45 percent of all infants born in the United States. The following benefits are provided to WIC participants: supplemental nutritious foods; nutrition education and counseling at WIC clinics; screening and referrals to other health, welfare, and social services.

WIC is not an entitlement program, as Congress does not set aside funds to allow every eligible individual to participate in the program. WIC is a federal grant program that Congress authorizes a specific amount of funds for each year.

WIC is administered at the federal level by FNS, by eighty-eight WIC state agencies, and through approximately forty-six thousand authorized retailers. WIC operates through two thousand local agencies in ten thousand clinic sites, in fifty state health departments, thirty-three Indian Tribal Organizations, American Samoa, District of Columbia, Guam, Puerto Rico, and the Virgin Islands.

Since a major goal of the WIC Program is to improve the nutritional status of infants, WIC mothers are encouraged to breastfeed their infants. WIC has historically promoted breastfeeding to all pregnant women as the optimal infant feeding choice, unless medically contraindicated. WIC mothers choosing to breastfeed are provided information through counseling and educational materials.

Breastfeeding mothers receive follow-up support through peer counselors. Breastfeeding mothers are eligible to participate in WIC longer than non-breastfeeding mothers. Mothers who exclusively breastfeed their infants receive an enhanced food package. Breastfeeding mothers can receive breast pumps, breast shells, or nursing supplements to help support the initiation and continuation of breastfeeding.

"Loving Support Makes Breastfeeding Work" is the WIC breastfeeding promotion campaign, which is national in scope and implemented at the state agency level. The goals of the campaign are to: encourage WIC participants to initiate and continue breastfeeding; increase referrals to WIC for breastfeeding support; increase general public acceptance and support of breastfeeding; and provide technical assistance to WIC state and local agency professionals in the promotion of breastfeeding. Helping women feel comfortable with breastfeeding, offering tips on how breastfeeding can work around a busy schedule, and the involvement of family and friends to make breastfeeding a success is important to the WIC program.

WIC breastfeeding goals are to:

❖ Increase breastfeeding initiation rates among WIC participants.

❖ Increase breastfeeding duration among WIC participants.

❖ Increase referrals to WIC for breastfeeding support.

❖ Increase general public acceptance and support of breastfeeding.

❖ Provide support and technical assistance to WIC state and local agencies in the promotion of breastfeeding.

Fathers Supporting Breastfeeding

Fathers Supporting Breastfeeding is an FNS project targeted to African American fathers, so that they may positively impact a mother's decision to breastfeed. The project is part of a continual effort to increase breastfeeding initiation and duration rates among African American women by involving fathers in breastfeeding promotion efforts.

Chapter Eleven

Resources for Further Support

Breastfeeding Support
African American Breastfeeding Alliance
Provides breastfeeding education and support. Offers Breastfeeding Peer Counselor Training. Consults on issues facing breastfeeding African American women. Offers free copies of *An Easy Guide to Breastfeeding for African American Women* and *The Love of Breastfeeding Your Baby*. Provides information on starting a chapter of AABA, and how to become a breast-feeding peer counselor or lactation consultant.
(877) 532-8535
www.aabaonline.com

Breastfeeding Legislation
Representative Carolyn B. Maloney, 14th Congressional District New York.
(202) 225-7944
www.house.gov/maloney/issues/breastfeeding
rep.carolyn.maloney@mail.house.gov

Healthy Mothers, Healthy Babies of Washington
Promoting, protecting, and supporting breastfeeding as a vital part of the

health and development of children and their families. Includes tools for working with your employer.
www.hmhbwa.org

La Leche League International
(847) 519-7730
www.lalecheleague.org

Mocha Moms
Support group for stay-at-home mothers of color. Offers support for mothers. Provides events for mothers, children, and families. Focuses on community service.
www.mochamoms.org

National Women's Health Information Center Breastfeeding Helpline
(800) 944-9662
www.WomansHealth.gov

Websites
www.4woman.gov/breastfeeding
www.bflrc.com
www.breastfeeding.com
www.breastfeedingtaskforla.org
www.gotmom.org
www.ilca.org
www.kellymom.org
www.mothering.com
www.promom.org

Breastfeeding Products and Breast Pumps

Avent
(800) 54-AVENT

Bailey
www.baileymed.com

Lansinoh, Inc.
www.lansinoh.com

Medela, Inc.
(800) 435-8316
www.medela.com

Motherwear
www.motherwear.com

Books

The Breastfeeding Answer Book
by La Leche League International, Nancy Mohrbacher, and Julie Stock
Available at most bookstores or www.amazon.com.

The Breastfeeding Book
by Dr. William and Martha Sears
Available at most bookstores or www.amazon.com.

Breastfeeding Facts over Fiction: Health Implications on the African American Community
by Mishawn Purnell-O'Neal
Available for purchase by calling (708) 488-1458 or email the author at mishawnpurnell@msn.com.

Breastfeeding Pure & Simple
by Gwen Gotsch
Available at most bookstores or www.amazon.com.

The Ultimate Breastfeeding Book of Answers:
The Most Comprehensive Problem/Solution Guide to Breastfeeding
by Dr. Jack Newman and Teresa Pitman
Available at most bookstores or www.amazon.com.

The Womanly Art of Breastfeeding
by La Leche League International
Available at most bookstores or www.amazon.com.

Appendix

Breastfeeding Laws by State

(From Summary of State Breastfeeding Legislation; reprinted with permission from *50 States Summary of Breastfeeding Laws*, www.ncsl.org/programs/health/breast50.htm. Copyright © 2004 by National Conference of State Legislatures)

Please note that new breastfeeding laws may have been passed since the printing of this book. You should check with your local government and online for an updated list.

Alaska

Alaska Stat. § 29.25.080 (1998) prohibits a municipality from enacting an ordinance that prohibits or restricts a woman breastfeeding a child in a public or private location where the woman and child are otherwise authorized to be. The law clarifies that "lewd conduct," "lewd touching," "immoral conduct," "indecent conduct," and similar terms do not include the act of a woman breastfeeding a child in a public or private location where the woman and child are otherwise authorized to be. (SB 297)

California

Cal. Civil Code § 210.5 (2000) allows the mother of a breastfed child to postpone jury duty for one year, and specifically eliminates the need for the mother to appear in court to request the postponement. The law also provides that the one-year period may be extended upon written request of the mother. [Chap. 266 (AB 1814)]

Cal. Health and Safety Code § 1647 (1999) declares that the procurement, processing, distribution, or use of human milk for the purpose of human consumption is considered to be a rendition of service rather than a sale of human milk. [Chap. 87 (AB 532)]

Cal. Assembly Concurrent Resolution 155 (1998) encourages the state and employers to support and encourage the practice of breastfeeding by striving to accommodate the needs of employees, and by ensuring that employees are provided with adequate facilities for breastfeeding and expressing milk for their children. The resolution memorializes the governor to declare by executive order that all state employees be provided with adequate facilities for breastfeeding and expressing milk.

Cal. Civil Code § 43.3 (1997) allows a mother to breastfeed her child in any location, public or private, except the private home or residence of another, where the mother and the child are otherwise authorized to be present. (AB 157)

Cal. Assembly Concurrent Resolution 95 (1996) proclaims the week of August 1 through 7, 1996, as Breastfeeding Awareness Week.

Cal. Health and Safety Code § 123360, 123365 (1995) requires the Department of Health Services to include in its public service campaign the promotion of mothers who breastfeed their infants. The law requires hospitals to make available a breastfeeding consultant or alternatively, provide information to the mother on where to receive breastfeeding information. (AB 973, AB 977)

Cal. Assembly Concurrent Resolution 41 (1995) proclaims August 1 through 7, 1995, Breastfeeding Awareness Week.

Colorado

CRS 25-6-301, 25-6-302 (2004) recognizes the benefits of breastfeeding and encourages mothers to breastfeed. The law also allows a mother to breastfeed in any place she has a right to be. (SB 88)

Connecticut

Conn. Public Act § 01-182 (2001) requires employers to provide reasonable time each day to an employee who needs to express breast milk for her infant child and to provide accommodations where an employee can express her milk in privacy. [HF 5656]

Conn. Gen. Stat. § 46a-64 (1997) prohibits places of public accommodation, resorts, or amusements from restricting or limiting the right of a mother to breastfeed her child. [P.A. 97-210]

Delaware

Del. Code Ann. tit. 31 § 310 (1997) entitles a mother to breastfeed her child in any location of a place of public accommodation wherein the mother is otherwise permitted. [71 Del. Laws, c. 10, § 1]

Florida

Fla. Senate Bill 170 (1999) creates certain offenses under the Children's Protective Act, and provides an exception for maternal breastfeeding.

Fla. Stat. § 383.016 (1994) authorizes a facility lawfully providing maternity services or newborn infant care to use the designation "baby-friendly" on its promotional materials. The facility must be in compliance with at least 80 percent of the requirements developed by the Department of Health in accordance with UNICEF and World Health Organization baby-friendly hospital initiatives. (SB 1668)

Fla. Stat. § 383.015 (1993) allows a mother to breastfeed in any public or private location. (HB 231) ct No. 922 (2002) changes the previous law, § 31-1-9, and inserts phrase: "The breastfeeding of a baby is an important and basic act of nurture which should be encouraged in the interests of maternal and child health. A mother may breastfeed her baby in any location where the mother and baby are otherwise authorized to be." (S.B. 221)

Ga. Code § 31-1-9 (1999) allows a mother to breastfeed in any location where she is otherwise authorized to be, provided that she "acts in a discreet and modest way." [Act 304 (SB 29)]

Ga. Code § 34-1-6 (1999) allows employers to provide daily, unpaid break time for a mother to express breast milk for her infant child. Employers may also be required to make a reasonable effort to provide a private location (other than a toilet stall) in close proximity to the workplace for this activity. The employer is not required to provide break time if to do so would unduly disrupt the workplace operations.

Hawaii

Hawaii Rev. Stat. § 367-3 (1999) requires the Hawaii Civil Rights Commission to collect, assemble, and publish data concerning instances of discrimination involving breastfeeding or expressing breast milk in the workplace. Prohibits employers to forbid an employee from expressing breast milk during any meal period or other break period. (HB 266)

Hawaii Rev. Stat. § 378-2 (1999) makes it discriminatory to deny the full and equal enjoyment of the goods, services, facilities, privileges, advantages, and accommodations of a place of public accommodations to a woman because she is breastfeeding a child. (HB 2774)

Idaho

Code 2-209 (1996) allows nursing mothers to postpone jury service until she is no longer nursing the child.

Illinois

Ill. P.A. 93-942 (2004) creates the Right to Breastfeed Act. Provides that a mother may breastfeed her baby in any location, public or private, where the mother is otherwise authorized to be; a mother who breastfeeds in a place of worship shall follow the appropriate norms within that place of worship. (SB 3211)

Ill. Law, P.A. 92-68 (2001) creates the Nursing Mothers in the Workplace Act, and requires that employers provide reasonable unpaid break time each day to employees who need to express breast milk. The law also requires employers to make reasonable efforts to provide a room or other location, other than a toilet stall, where an employee can express her milk in privacy. (SB 542).

Ill. Rev. Stat. ch. 20 § 2310/55.84 (1997) allows the Department of Public Health to conduct an information campaign for the general public to promote breastfeeding of infants by their mothers. The law allows the department to include the information in a brochure that shares other information with the general public, and is distributed free of charge. [P.A. 90–244]

Ill. Rev. Stat. ch. 720 § 5/11-9 (1995) clarifies that breastfeeding of infants is not an act of public indecency. (SB 190)

3-35-6 allows a woman to breastfeed her infant anywhere that the ⅃lows her to be. (HB 1510)

Iowa

Code § 607A.5 (1994) allows a woman to be excused from jury service if she submits written documentation verifying, to the court's satisfaction, that she is the mother of a breastfed child and is responsible for the daily care of the child.

Iowa Code § 135.30A (2002) a woman may breastfeed the woman's own child in any public place where the woman's presence is otherwise authorized.

Louisiana

La. House Concurrent Resolution 35 (2002) establishes a joint study of requiring insurance coverage for outpatient lactation support for new mothers.

LRS 51. 2247.1 (2001) states that a mother may breastfeed her baby in any place of public accommodation, resort, or amusement, and clarifies that breastfeeding is not a violation of law. (HB 377)

LRS 46. 1409 B 5 prohibits any child care facility from discriminating against breastfed babies. (HB 233)

Maine

Me. Rev. Stat. Ann. tit. 5, § 4634 (2001) amends the Maine Human Rights Act to declare that a mother has the right to breastfeed her baby in any location, whether public or private, as long as she is otherwise authorized to be in that location. [Public Law No. 206 (LD 1396)]

Me. Rev. Stat. Ann. tit. 19-a § 1653 (1999) requires the court, in making an award of parental rights and responsibilities with respect to a child, to apply the standard of the best interest of the child. In making decisions regarding the child's residence and parent-child contact, the court must consider primarily the safety and well-being of the child, and consider whether the child is under one year of age, and being breastfed. [Public Law No. 702 (HB 2774)]

Maryland

Md. Laws, Chap. 369 (2003) permits a woman to breastfeed her infant in any public or private place, and prohibits anyone from restricting or limiting this right. (SB223)

Michigan

Mich. Comp. Laws §§ 41.181,67.1aa, and 117.4i (1994) states that public nudity laws do not apply to a woman breastfeeding a child.

Minnesota

Minn. Laws, Chap. 269 (2000) allows a nursing mother, upon request, to be excused from jury service if she is not employed outside of her home, and if she is responsible for the daily care of the child. (HF 1865)

Minn.Stat. § 181.939 (1998) requires employers to provide daily unpaid break time for a mother to express breast milk for her infant child. Employers are also required to make a reasonable effort to provide a private location (other than a toilet stall) in close proximity to the workplace for this activity. (SB 2751)

Missouri

Mo. Rev. Stat. § 191.915 (1999) requires hospitals and ambulatory surgical centers to provide new mothers with information on breastfeeding, the

…ne child, and information on local breastfeeding support groups …sultation. The law requires physicians who provide obstetrical or …ological consultation to inform patients about the postnatal benefits …oreastfeeding. The law requires the Department of Health to provide …and distribute written information on breastfeeding and the health benefits to the child. (SB 8)

Mo. Rev. Stat. § 191.918 (1999) allows a mother, with as much discretion as possible, to breastfeed her child in any public or private location.

Montana

Mont. Code Ann. § 50-19-501 (1999) states that the breastfeeding of a child in any location, public or private, can not be considered a nuisance, indecent exposure, sexual conduct, or obscenity. (SB 398)

Nebraska

Neb. Rev. Stat. §25-1601-4 (2004) states that a nursing mother is excused from jury duty until she is no longer breastfeeding; nursing mother must file qualification form supported by certificate from her physician requesting exemption.

Nevada

Rev. Stat. § 201.232 (1995) states that the breastfeeding of a child in any location, public or private, is not considered a violation of indecent-exposure laws. (SB 317)

New Hampshire

Rev. Stat. Ann. § 121:1, et seq. (1999) states that breastfeeding does not constitute indecent exposure, and that limiting or restricting a mother's right to breastfeed is discriminatory. [HB 441]

New Jersey
N.J. Rev. Stat. § 26:4B–4 (1997) entitles a mother to breastfeed her baby in any location, including public accommodations, resorts, or amusements. Failure to comply with the law may result in a fine.

New Mexico
Stat. Ann. § 28-20-1 (1999) permits a mother to breastfeed her child in any public or private location where she is otherwise authorized to be. (SB 545)

New York
N.Y. Civil Rights Law § 79-e (1994) permits a mother to breastfeed her child in any public or private location. (SB 3999)

North Carolina
N.C. Gen. Stat. § 14-190.9 (1993) states that a woman is allowed to breastfeed in any public or private location, and she is not in violation of indecent exposure laws. (HB 1143)

Oklahoma
2004 OK Laws, Chap. 332 allows a mother to breastfeed her child in any location that she is authorized to be, and exempts her from the crimes and punishments listed in the penal code of the state of Oklahoma. Additionally, mothers who are breastfeeding can request to be exempt from service as jurors. (HB 2102)

Oregon
Or. Rev. Stat. § 109.001 (1999) allows a woman to breastfeed in a public place. (SB 744)

Or. Rev. Stat. § 10.050 (1999) excuses a woman from acting as a juror

.s breastfeeding a child. A request from the woman must be
.ting. (SB 1304)

...e Island

.I. Gen. Laws § 23-13.2-1 (2003) calls for employers to provide a safe private place for an employee to breastfeed her child and express breast milk. (HB 5507/SB 151)

R.I. Gen. Laws § 23-72-1 (2001) requires the Department of Health to prepare a consumer mercury alert notice. The notice shall explain the danger of eating mercury-contaminated fish to women who are pregnant or breastfeeding their children.

(HB 6112)R.I. Gen. Laws § 11-45-1 (1998) excludes mothers engaged in breastfeeding from disorderly conduct laws. (HB 8103, SB 2319)

South Dakota
SD § 22-22-24.1 (2002) exempts mothers who are breastfeeding from indecency laws.

Tennessee
Tenn. Code Ann. § 50-1-305 (1999) requires employers to provide daily unpaid break time for a mother to express breast milk for her infant child. Employers are also required to make a reasonable effort to provide a private location (other than a toilet stall) in close proximity to the workplace for this activity. (SB 1856)

Texas
Tex. Health Code § 161.071 (2001) calls for the Department of Health to establish minimum guidelines for the procurement, processing, distribution, or use of human milk by donor milk banks. (HB 391)

Tex. Health Code Ann. § 165.001, et seq. (1995) authorizes a woman to breastfeed her child in any location, and provides for the use of a "mother-friendly" designation for employers who have policies supporting work site breastfeeding. (HB 340, HB 359)

Utah

Utah Code Ann. § 17-15-25 (1995) states that city and county governing bodies may not inhibit a woman's right to breastfeed in public.

Utah Code Ann. § 76-10-1229.5 (1995) states that a breastfeeding woman is not in violation of any obscene or indecent exposure laws. (H.B. 262)

Vermont

Vt. Acts, Chap. No. 117 (2002) finds that breastfeeding a child is an important, basic, and natural act of nurture that should be encouraged in the interest of enhancing maternal, child, and family health. The law allows a mother to breastfeed her child in any place of public accommodation in which the mother and child would otherwise have a legal right to be. The law directs the Human Rights Commission to develop and distribute materials that provide information regarding a woman's legal right to breastfeed her child in a place of public accommodation. (S.B. 156)

Virginia

Va. Code 2.2-1147.1 (2002) guarantees a woman the right to breastfeed her child on any property owned, leased, or controlled by the state. The bill also stipulates that childbirth and related medical conditions specified in the Virginia Human Rights Act include activities of lactation, including breastfeeding and expression of milk by a mother for her child. (H.B. 1264)

HJ 145 (2002) Encourages employers to recognize the benefits of breast-feeding and to provide unpaid break time and appropriate space for employees to breastfeed or express milk.

Va. Code § 18.2-387 (1994) exempts mothers engaged in breastfeeding from indecent exposure laws.

Va. Chapter No. 195 (2005) Provides that a mother who is breastfeed-ing a child may be exempted from jury duty upon her request. The mother need not be "necessarily and personally responsible for a child or children 16 years of age or younger requiring continuous care…during normal court hours" as the existing statute provides.

Washington

Wash. Revised Code § 9A.88.010 (2001) states that the act of breastfeeding or expressing breast milk is not indecent exposure. (HB 1590)

Wash. Revised Code § 43.70 (2001) allows any employer (governmen-tal and private) to use the designation of "infant-friendly" on its promo-tional materials if the employer follows certain requirements. [Chap. 88]

Wisconsin

Wis. Stat. §§ 944.17(3), 944.20(2) and 948.10(2) (1995) provide that breastfeeding mothers are not in violation of criminal statutes of indecent or obscene exposure. (AB 154)

Wyoming

Wyo. House Joint Resolution 5 (2003) encourages breastfeeding and rec-ognizes the importance of breastfeeding to maternal and child health. The resolution also commends employers, both in the public and private sec-tors, who provide accommodations for breastfeeding mothers.

A Sampling of Workplace Laws Promoting Breastfeeding around the World

Argentina: Working mothers of nursing babies have the right to two daily half-hour breaks for breastfeeding during work time for one year after the baby is born.

Canada: In British Columbia, employers are required to accommodate women who wish to breastfeed children during work hours, unless their absence would cause undue hardship.

Egypt: For eighteen months after delivery, women are granted two daily breaks of not less than half an hour each. Breaks may be combined if the female employee so desires. These breaks are in addition to the normal breaks granted to employees generally, and do not result in any reduction of pay.

France: Nursing mothers are allowed to take two hour breaks from work. Nursing rooms and breastfeeding rooms must be provided by the employer.

Israel: For four months after delivery, a nursing mother may be absent from work one hour a day, as long as she is employed in a full-time job. The employee will not get deducted pay for this hour absence.

Italy: Full-time working women are allowed two paid, one-hour breaks to breastfeed. A woman who works six hours is entitled to a one-hour break for breastfeeding, and it can be split up into two half-hour breaks.

Japan: A full-time employee is granted two thirty-minute breaks a day in addition to set break periods. Part-time employees are allowed one thirty-minute break. The breaks are paid if there is a collective agreement in the workplace to pay for the breaks.

Mozambique: Maternity leave is only for two months, but two half-hour paid nursing breaks are provided during the workday for up to six months.

Norway: Working women are allowed two hours daily to breastfeed at work, and 99 percent of mothers are still breastfeeding after six weeks. (In contrast, according to a 1995 law review article, only 40 percent in England and 12 percent in Northern Ireland, where no such policies are in place.)

People's Republic of China: Provides two thirty-minute breaks per working shift for nursing infants up to age one, establishment of health clinics, breastfeeding rooms, and child care centers.

Russia: Nursing mothers are granted thirty-minute breaks at least every three hours. Breaks for a nursing child are included in work time and shall be paid according to the nursing mother's average earnings.

Sweden: A woman can take breaks to breastfeed her child as she wishes.

Tunisia: For nine months after delivery, a woman employee has two paid half-hour breaks in addition to the normal break times to breastfeed. Employees are required to provide breastfeeding rooms to their employees.

Turkey: Breastfeeding mothers are allowed two forty-five-minute periods to nurse. These periods are considered work hours.

Bibliography

American Academy of Pediatrics. *Breastfeeding Policy Statement: Breastfeeding and the Use of Human Milk Pediatrics*. Vol. 115 No. 2. February 2005.

Antolini, K Lane. *Negotiating Motherhood in the Antebellum South*. The University of Illinois Graduate Symposium on Women's and Gender History. 2003.

Baby-Friendly USA. *The Ten Steps to Successful Breastfeeding for Hospitals*. The Baby-Friendly Hospital Initiative. Massachusetts, USA.

Burby, L. *101 Reasons to Breastfeed*. ProMom, Inc. www.promom.org. May 2005.

Follett, R. *Heat, Sex and Sugar: Pregnancy and Childbearing in the Slave Quarters*. Journal of Family History. Vol. 28 No. 4. October 2003. 510-539.

Giugliani, ERJ. Bronner, Y. Caiaffa, WT. Vogelhut, J. Witter, FR. Perman, JA. "Are Fathers Prepared to Encourage Their Partners to Breastfeed?" *Acta Paediatra* 83:1127-31. 1994.

Haines, MR. Preston, SH. *Fatal Years: Child Mortality in Late Nineteenth Century America*. 26-29.

Hollister Incorporated. *Ameda Breastfeeding Guide*. USA, 2000.

La Leche League International. *Breastfeeding Peer Counselor Program Curriculum*. 1995.

MacClancy, J. "The Milk Tie." *Anthropology of Food*. Vol.1. Oxford Brooks University. 2003.

Medela. *Breastfeeding Information Guide: Breastfeeding Tips and Products*. USA, 2002.

Neifert, M. *Supporting Breastfeeding Mothers as They Return to Work*. American Academy of Pediatrics. 2000.

Riordan, J. Auerbach. K. *Breastfeeding and Human Lactation*. Jones and Bartlett Publishers. 1998. 2nd Edition.

Sears, S. Sears, M. *The Breastfeeding Book: Everything You Need to Know About Nursing Your Child From Birth Through Weaning*. Little, Brown and Company. 2000.

Thomas, VG. "The Psychology of Black Women: Studying Women's Lives in Context." *Journal of Black Psychology*. Vol. 30 No. 3. August 2004. 286-306.

U.S. Department of Health and Human Services Office on Women's Health. *HHS Blueprint for Action on Breastfeeding*. USDHHS, Office on Women's Health. Washington, DC. 2000.

U.S. Department of Health and Human Services. *Report of the Surgeon General's Workshop on Breastfeeding and Human Lactation*. USDHHS, HRSA, DHHS. Rockville, MD. No. HRS-D-MC 84-2. 1984.

UNICEF/WHO. *Innocenti Declaration on the Protection, Promotion and Support of Breastfeeding*. UNICEF and WHO. Florence, Italy. 1990.

United States Breastfeeding Committee. *Breastfeeding in the United States: A National Agenda*. US Department of Health and Human Services, Health Resources and Services Administration, Maternal and Child Health Bureau. Rockville, MD. 2001.

Young, M. Breastfeeding, *What's the Big Deal. Recapturing the Breastfeeding Tradition: The State of Breastfeeding in the African American Community*. Howard University Hospital. September 2003.

Index

A

AA (arachidonic acid), 33
AABA (African American Breastfeeding Alliance), 18, 208–212, 233
acute respiratory disease, 90
African American Breastfeeding Alliance (AABA), 18, 208–212, 233
alcohol abuse, 57
anorexia nervosa, 57
anxiety, 11
allergies, 89
Araujo-Rouse, Liza, 192–196
asthma, 3–5, 88

B

Baby-Friendly Hospital Initiative (BFHI), 212–214
Baby-Friendly USA, 213–214
Barber, Noel, 102–103
barriers to breastfeeding, 79–96
    culture, 80–81
    education and support, lack of, 82–84
    infant formula, 86–87
    inner doubts, 84–86
    myths, 81–82
BFHI (Baby-Friendly Hospital Initiative), 212–214
Blueprint for Action, 224–229
bottle, introducing, 124–126
bottles, 165–166
bowel movements, baby's, 67–69
Brandy, 183
breasts
    abscess, 57

alveoli, 31
areola, 17, 25–31
    ducts, 32
    montgomery glands, 17
    nipples, 17, 25–31, 163–164
    sinus, 31
breast cancer, 6–7
breastfeeding
    and breast size, 16
    and exercise, 168
    and fathers, 97–118
    and pregnancy, 65
    and slavery, 171–177
    and surgery, 166
    as birth control, 12–13
    barriers to, 79–96
    benefits for employer, 121–124
    duration of, 168
    football hold, 26
    how it works, 29–33
    how to, 23–33
    informing hospital staff, 20
    lying down, 27
    on demand, 162
    post-slavery, 178–181
    state guidelines for, 206–207, 237–248
    twins, 166
    world guidelines for, 249–250
breastfeeding, common concerns and solutions, 41–77
    allergies, family history of, 53
    breast changes, 50–51
    breast surgery, previous, 50
    depression, mild, 52
    disability, 50

engorgement, 43–45, 57
excessive fatigue, maternal, 51
lactation failure, previous, 50
mastitis, 46–48
nipples, flat or inverted, 50
plugged ducts, 45–46
prescription drugs, 52–53, 61–63
sore nipples, 41–43
thrush, 48–49
breastfeeding-friendly companies, 135
breast milk
    antibodies in, 35
    baby getting enough, 36–39, 66–74
    digestibility, 8
    expressing by hand, 38
    eye coordination, 9
    immune system, 8–9
    increasing, 72–74
    ingredients in, 33–35
    IQ, 8
    labeling stored, 132
    nutrients in, 7, 33–35
    pump, how to, 135
    storing, 130–132
    supply, concern about, 56–57
    teeth, 9
    thawing, 130–132
breast pump, 126–127, 235
bulimia, 57

C

cancers, childhood, 90–91
cardiovascular disease, 92–93
chicken pox exposure, 57
child-care provider, 136–139
chronic diseases, childhood, 91
cleft palate, 58
colic, 54–55, 162

colostrum, 8, 17, 35
Covin, Michael, 99–100
c-section, 27
CT scan, 64, 159

D

dads and breastfeeding, 97–118
dads concerns, 112–113
dads, facts for, 114–115
dehydration, 57–58
Department of Health and Human
    Services (DHHS), 217–220
DHA (docosahexaenoic acid), 33
DHHS (Department of Health and
    Human Services), 217–220
diabetes, 91–92
diarrhea, 53–54, 65, 164–165
drug use, history of, 57

E

Eades-Jones, Desireé, 202–203
employer, sample letter to, 127–130
employment, returning to, 119–139
engorgement, 43–45, 57

F

fathers and breastfeeding, 97–118
fathers concerns, 112–113
fathers, facts for, 114–115
Fathers Supporting Breastfeeding, 231
fenugreek, 56–57
football hold, 26
formula feeding, risks of, 88–96
    acute respiratory disease, 90
    allergies, 89
    asthma, 88

cancers, childhood, 90–91
cardiovascular disease, 92–93
chronic diseases, childhood, 91
cognitive development, reduced, 89
diabetes, 91–92
gastrointestinal infections, 94
mortality, increased, 94–95
obesity, childhood, 5–6, 93
otitis media and ear infections, 95
side effects of environmental
contaminants, 95–96
frenulum, short, 58

G

gastrointestinal infections, 94

H

Healthy People 2010, 209
hepatitis B, 57
Hill, Lauryn, 183
HIV positive, 13, 57, 63

I

illness, maternal, 63
ILO (International Labor Organization),
205–206
INFACT Canada, 88–96
Innocenti Declaration, 218
International Labor Organization (ILO),
205–206

J

jaundice, 53, 65–66
Johnson, Magic, 183
Jordan, Michael, 183

L

lactose intolerance, 8
La Leche League (LLL), 18, 214, 234
Lansinoh, 199, 211
latch, breaking baby's, 29
latching on, 27
LLL (La Leche League), 18, 214, 234
Long, Dr. Sahira, 198–201

M

mammograms, 64
mastitis, 46–48, 57, 64
maternal illness, 63
maternity leave, 205–206
measles exposure, 57
McIlwaine, Michelle, 196–198
Mocha Moms, 18, 184, 234
MRI scan, 64, 159
myths, breastfeeding, 141–169

N

neurological impairment, 58–59
Newman, Dr. Jack, 61, 159, 236
nipple confusion, 22, 163

O

obesity, childhood, 5–6, 93
on-demand breastfeeding, 162
otitis media, 95
oxytocin, 9, 12, 32

P

Peete, Holly Robinson, 183
physician, when to contact, 57–59
pituitary gland, 32

postpartum psychosis, 57
postpartum thyroiditis, 64
post-slavery breastfeeding, 178–181
premature baby, 54, 59
prescription drugs, 52–53, 61–63
prolactin, 12, 32
pump, how to, 135

R

respiratory illness in baby, 65

S

scales and weights, 73
schedule, restrictive, 56
self-actualization, 188–189
self-empowerment, 187–188
self-esteem, 189–190
Sherrod, Leslie, 190–192
SIDS (Sudden Infant Death Syndrome),
  2–3
slavery, 171–177
Smith, Jada Pinkett, 183
solid foods, 74–77
Special Supplemental Nutrition Program
  for Women, Infants, and Children
  (WIC),18, 209, 229–231
statistics, xii–xiii, 181–184, 206
Sudden Infant Death Syndrome (SIDS),
  2–3
Surgeon General's Workshop on
  Breastfeeding and Human Lactation
  (1984), 220–222

T

twins, 166, 183

U

UNICEF, 215–216
United States Breastfeeding Committee
  (USBC), 216–217, 222–223
urination, baby's, 69–70
USBC (United States Breastfeeding
  Committee), 216–217, 222–223

V

vomiting, 53–54, 65

W

Walker-Gordon Milk Laboratory, 180
weaning, 59–60, 176
weight loss, 9, 59
weight, slow gain of, 54
wet nursing, 171, 174–177
WHO (World Health Organization), 215
WIC (Special Supplemental Nutrition
  Program for Women, Infants, and
  Children), 18, 209, 229–231
work, returning to, 119–139
World Health Organization (WHO), 215

X

X-rays, 64, 159

About the Author

Kathi Barber is a certified lactation educator and counselor, and is the Founder and Executive Director of the African American Breastfeeding Alliance (AABA), a national nonprofit organization that educates African American women and the professionals who serve them about the importance of breastfeeding African American babies. She is a sought-after speaker, and regularly travels across the country to conduct workshops and lecture about breastfeeding and African American women. She is a consultant with the United States Department of Health and Human Services Office on Women's Health, and is a member of the United States Breastfeeding Committee. Her work for AABA has been featured in the *Washington Post, Ebony Magazine, USA Today,* and the *Chicago Tribune.*

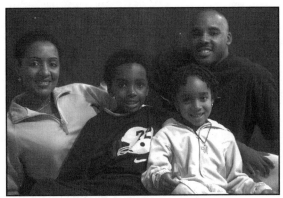

Author photo © 2004 Andrew Foster